The Elbow

Springer
Berlin
Heidelberg
New York
Barcelona
Budapest
Hong Kong
London
Milan
Paris
Santa Clara
Singapore
Tokyo

W. Rüther (Ed.)

The Elbow

Endoprosthetic Replacement and Non-Endoprosthetic Procedures

With 131 Figures and 19 Tables

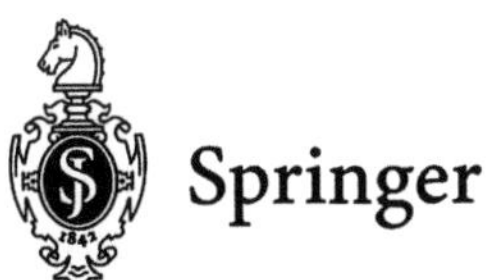

Springer

Prof. Dr.med. W. Rüther
Orthopädische Klinik
Heinrich-Heine-Universität
Moorenstr. 5
40225 Düsseldorf
Germany

ISBN-13: 978-3-642-79741-5   e-ISBN-13: 978-3-642-79739-2
DOI: 10.1007/978-3-642-79739-2

Library of Congress Cataloging-in-Publication Data. The elbow:endoprosthetic replacement and non-endoprosthetic procedures/W. Rüther (ed.). p. cm. Includes bibliographical references. ISBN-13: 978-3-642-79741-5   1. Elbow—Surgery. 2. Total elbow replacement. I. Rüther, Wolfgang. [DNLM: 1. Elbow—surgery. 2. Elbow Joint—surgery. 3. Prosthesis. 4. Arthroplasty. WE 820 E3837 1995] RD558.E437 1995 617.5'74—dc20 DNLM/DLC for Library of Congress 95–31211

Cover design: Springer-Verlag, Design & Production

Typesetting: Best-set Typesetter Ltd., Hong Kong

SPIN: 10129733   24/3135/SPS – 5 4 3 2 1 0 – Printed on acid free paper

Preface

Concepts in total elbow arthroplasty have changed within the past few years. Various elbow implants are now available which differ mainly regarding constraint, transmission of load between the implant and the bone, fixation of components, and required surgical techniques. In general, according to current clinical experience endoprosthetic replacement can be offered to patients with painful arthritic or posttraumatic elbow. However, the question arises as to whether the classical method of resection arthroplasty still has a role in modern surgery, particular for arthritis. This is of special interest because resection arthroplasties have proved to be most useful in the elbow. New surgical techniques such as distraction arthroplasty indicate that there is a need for nonendoprosthetic procedures in advanced destruction of the elbow.

In March 1994 renowned specialists and designers of approved endoprostheses were invited to a 3-day symposium in Düsseldorf, Germany, to present their personal experience and to update the information in the field of elbow arthroplasty. The contributions addressed issues regarding implant arthroplasties and different types of non-endoprosthetic procedures. The surgical demonstrations in cadaver specimens emphasized the significance of surgical details and the necessity of skillful surgical technique. The oral presentations, which are contained in this book, encouraged discussions and illustrated the convergence and divergence in various procedures. Nearly 150 participants from all over Europe attended this meeting.

We thank Mrs. J. Hemmers for her excellent secretarial assistance. We acknowledge Mrs. H. Kraffczyk, Dr. P. Dann, Dr. B. Fink, Dr. M. Pössel, Dr. T. Schneider, Dr. M. Strauss, Dr. L. Wiesner, and Dr. S. Zeisberger for their efforts in the preparation of this meeting, and the generous cooperation of many manufacturers and companies that provided financial support. Grateful acknowledgment, moreover, is given to Prof. Dr. K.-P. Schulitz for his support and the opportunity to organize this meeting with in the curriculum "Frühjahrssymposion der Orthopädischen Klinik, Düsseldorf".

Düsseldorf 1995 W. Rüther

Contents

Complications and Salvage Procedures

List of Contributors

Arens, S.
Klinik und Poliklinik für Unfallchirurgie, Sigmund-Freud-Str. 25,
53105 Bonn-Venusberg, Germany

Bähler, A.
Schulthess Klinik, Neumünsterallee 3, 8008 Zürich, Switzerland

Baltzer, A.
Orthopedic Clinic, University of Düsseldorf, Moorenstr. 5,
40225 Düsseldorf, Germany

Bretschneider, W.
Department of Orthopedics, University of Vienna,
Währinger Gürtel 18–20, 1090 Vienna, Austria

Figgie, M.P.
The Hospital for Special Surgery, Cornell University Medical College,
New York, NY 10021, USA

Gschwend, N.
Schulthess Klinik, Neumünsterallee 3, 8008 Zürich, Switzerland

Hansis, M.
Klinik und Poliklinik für Unfallchirurgie, Sigmund-Freud-Str. 25,
53105 Bonn-Venusberg, Germany

Inglis, A.E.
Center for Advanced Orthopaedic Surgery, 1725 York Avenue,
New York, NY 10128, USA

Jantea, C.
Orthopedic Clinic, University of Düsseldorf, Moorenstr. 5,
40225 Düsseldorf, Germany

Kerschbaumer, F.
Department of Surgery of Rheumatoid Arthritis,
University of Frankfurt, Marienburgstr. 2,
60528 Frankfurt, Germany

Kudo, H.
Chief of Orthopaedic Section, Sagamihara National Hospital,
Sakuradi, Sagamihara City, Kanagawa, Japan

Landor, I.
Prednosta Ortopedicka Klinika, Na Bojisti 1, 12821 Praha 2,
Czech Republic

Ljung, P.
Department of Orthopedics, University Hospital, 22185 Lund,
Sweden

Morrey, B.F.
Department of Orthopedics, Mayo Clinic, Rochester, MN 55905, USA

O'Driscoll, S.W.
Department of Orthopedics, Mayo Clinic, Rochester, MN 55905, USA

Richtr, M.
Prednosta Ortopedicka Klinika, Na Bojisti 1, 12821 Praha 2,
Czech Republic

Risung, F.
Department of Rheuma Surgery, Betanien Hospital,
3722 Skien, Norway

Rüther, W.
Orthopedic Clinic, University of Düsseldorf, Moorenstr. 5,
40225 Düsseldorf, Germany

Rydholm, U.
Department of Orthopedics, University Hospital, 22185 Lund,
Sweden

Scheier, H.
Schulthess Klinik, Neumünsterallee 3, 8008 Zürich, Switzerland

Simmen, B.
Schulthess Klinik, Neumünsterallee 3, 8008 Zürich, Switzerland

Sosna, A.
Prednosta Ortopedicke Klinika 1 LF UK, Na Bojisti 1,
12821 Praha 2, Czech Republic

Stanley, D.
Department of Orthopaedics, Northern General Hospital Trust,
Herries Road, Sheffield S5 7AU, England

Stiles, P.J.
Royal Country Hospital, 5, Fairway Merraow, Guildford GUI ZXG

Tillmann, K.
Orthopädische Abteilung in der Rheuma Klinik Bad Bramstedt
GmbH, Postfach 1448, 24572 Bad Bramstedt, Germany

Wanivenhaus, A.
Department of Orthopedics, University of Vienna,
Währinger Gürtel 18–20, 1090 Vienna, Austria

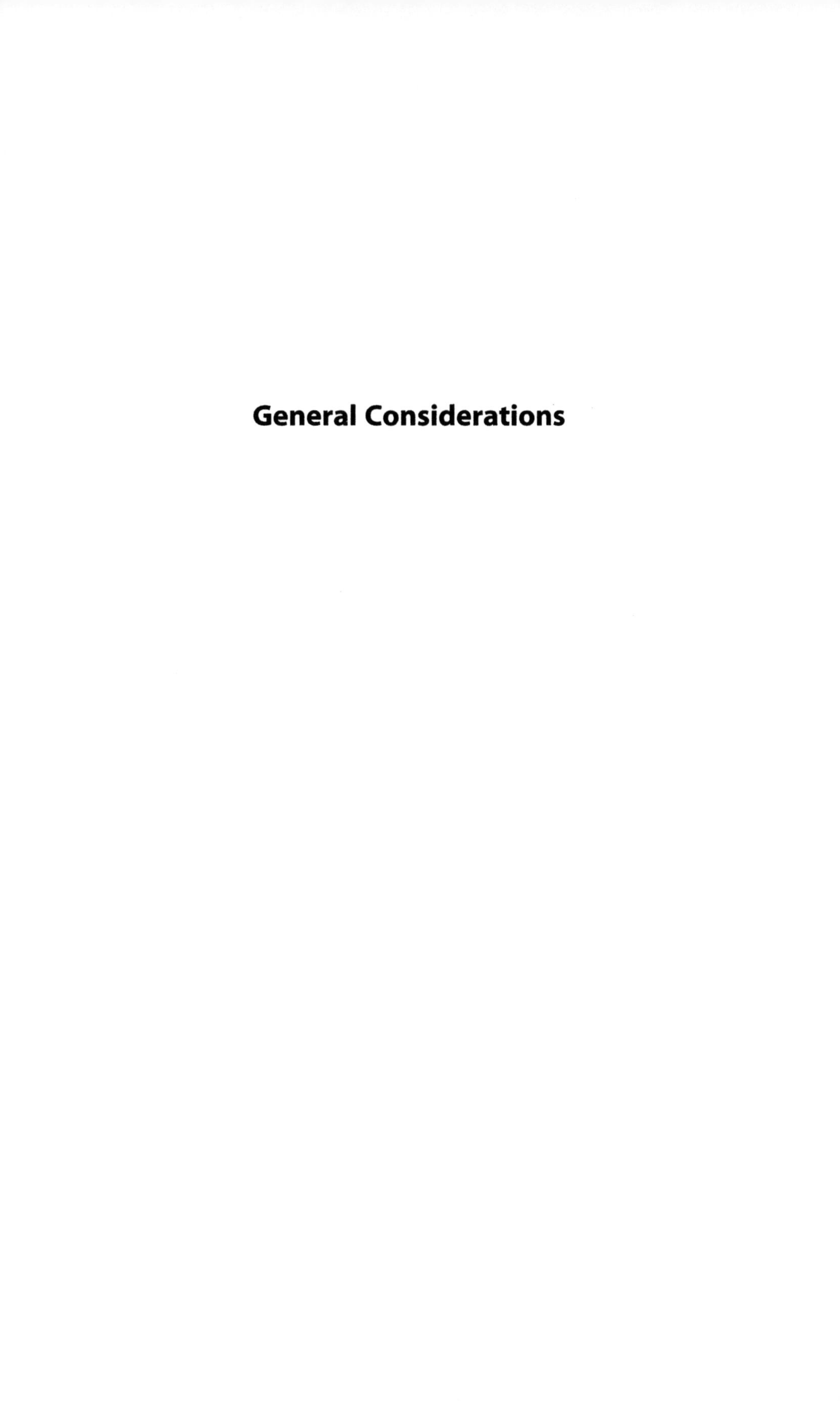

General Considerations

Surgical Treatment of the Rheumatoid Elbow

F. Kerschbaumer

General Considerations

The elbow joint has a central role regarding the function of the upper extremity. There is general agreement that ankylosis of the elbow joint as well as gross instability may lead to a major impairment of the whole upper extremity. Both the ankylotic and the flail elbow may be the result of juvenile or adult forms of rheumatoid arthritis (Figs. 1, 2).

The prevalence of elbow involvement in rheumatoid conditions varies between 39% and 72% [10, 19, 27, 31], depending on the type of rheumatoid disease. The natural course of elbow arthritis first shows juxta-articular porosis and slight narrowing of the joint space and later erosive changes and deformity of the proximal radioulnar, humeroradial, and humeroulnar joint with valgus instability. When talking about the elbow, we must remember that our concern is not only the joint, but the whole anatomic elbow region, including nerves, tendons, and vessels.

Entrapment Neuropathy

Entrapment neuropathy of the median, radial, and ulnar nerve has been well described for patients with rheumatoid disease [18, 20, 22, 24–26]. Three clinical examples may show the impact of these changes:

1. A male patient with seronegative pauciarticular arthritis was admitted with palsy of the long thumb flexor and paresis of the index long flexor. After electroneurological confirmation of the so-called Kiloh-Nevin syndrome, a decompression of the anterior interosseous nerve and resection of a small antecubital cyst was performed (Figs. 3, 4). Eight weeks later, a muscular force grade IV was obtained in both thumb and index finger.
2. A female patient with an unstable and destructed elbow complained of weakness in finger spreading. Froment's sign was positive. During surgery, compression of the ulnar nerve by medial osteophytes was found. After implantation of a semiconstrained total elbow prosthesis (GSB) and transposition of the ulnar nerve according to Eaton, a slow recovery of the muscular force was achieved after 6 months (Figs. 5, 6).

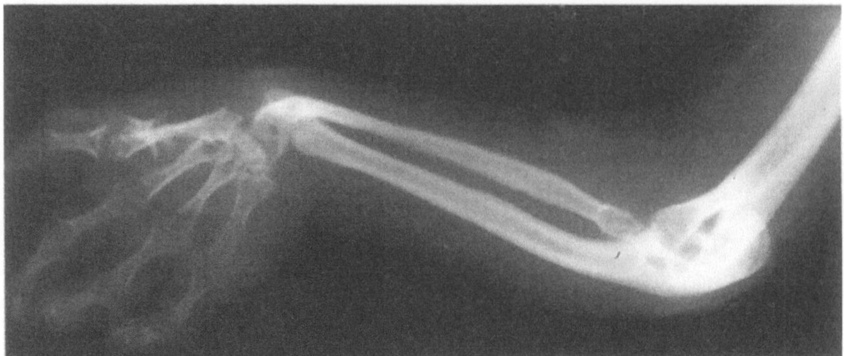

Fig. 1. Ankylotic elbow in juvenile rheumatoid arthrosis

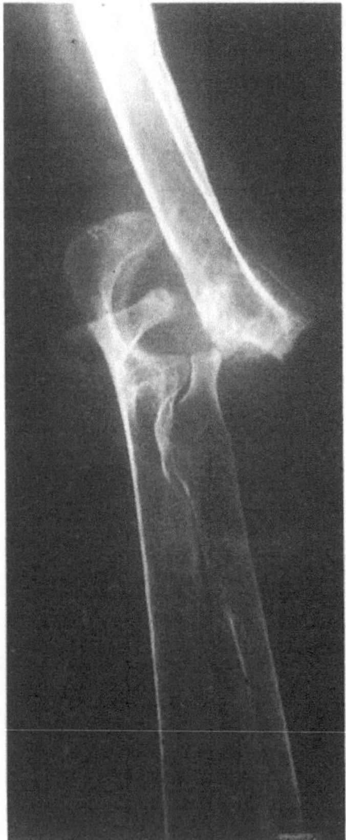

Fig. 2. Flail elbow in adult rheumatoid arthrosis (from [14])

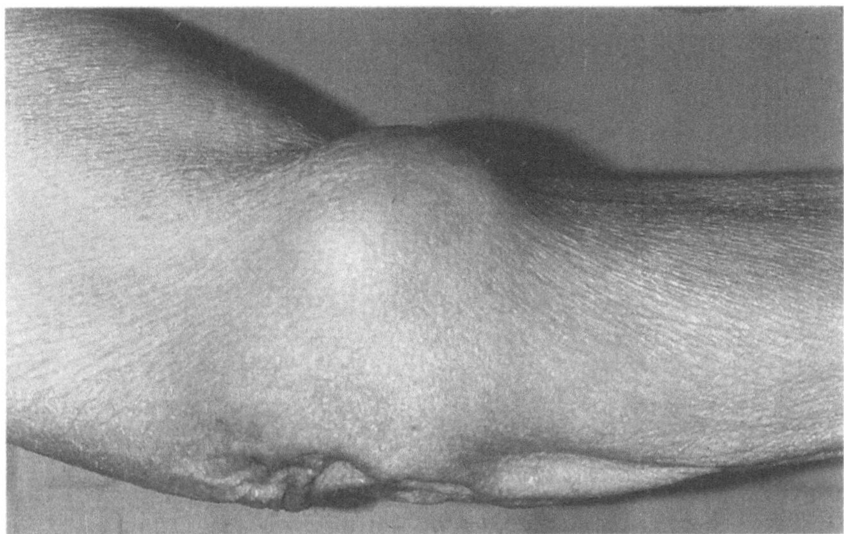

Fig. 3. Antecubital cyst

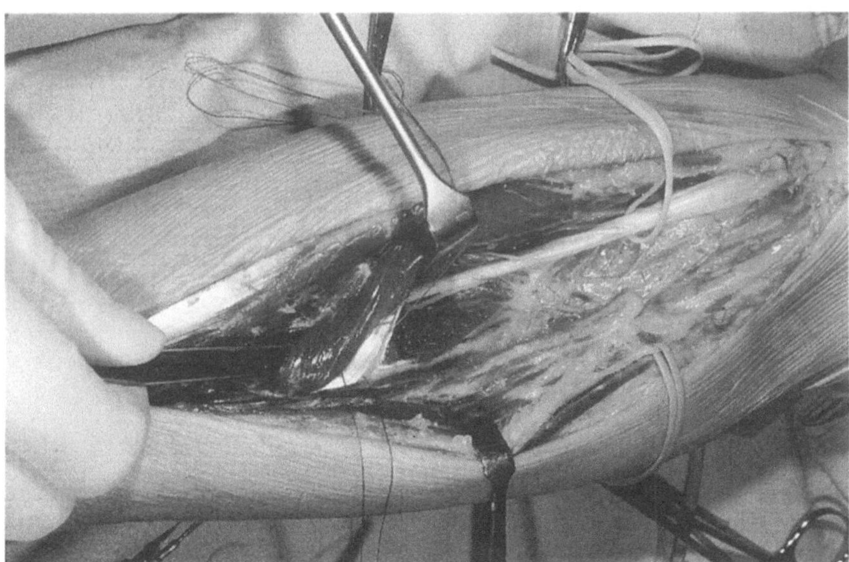

Fig. 4. Decompression of anterior interosseus nerve after cyst resection

3. A young woman with rheumatoid arthritis was admitted for extensor tendon reconstruction of the right hand. In fact, no tendon rupture was evident, but there was palsy of the fourth and fifth finger extensor as well as extensor carpi ulnaris tendons (Figs. 7, 8). The preoperative sonography showed a large synovitis with compression of the radial nerve. Twelve weeks after radial head resection, synovectomy, and decompression, active finger extension was possible (Figs. 9, 10)

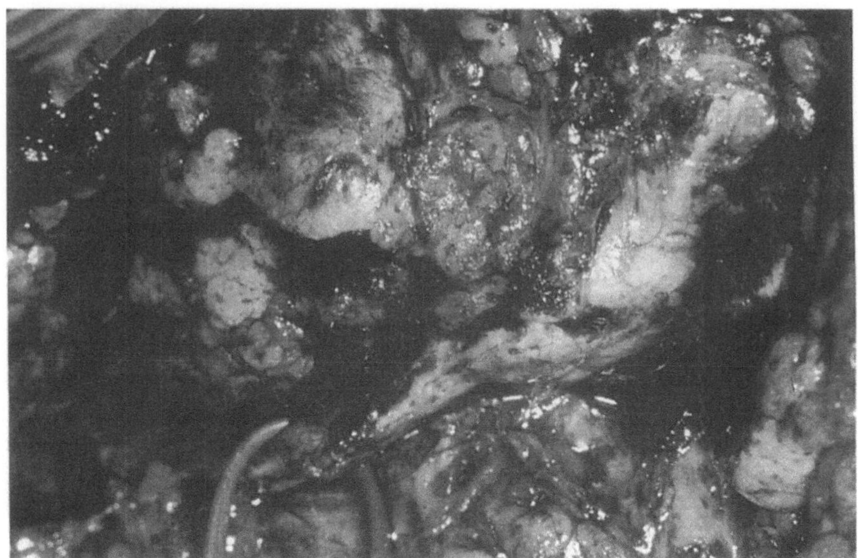

Fig. 5. Ulnar nerve neuropathy after decompression

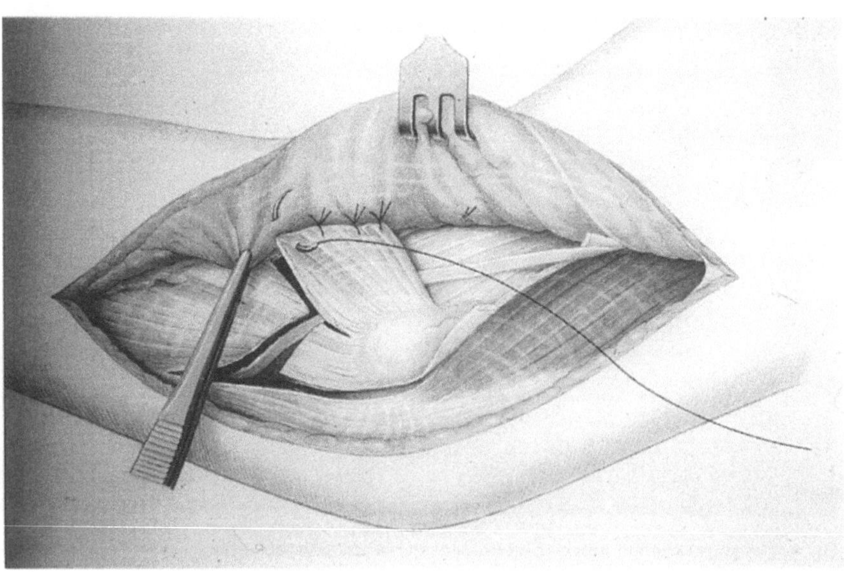

Fig. 6. Anterior transposition of ulnar nerve according to Eaton (from [15])

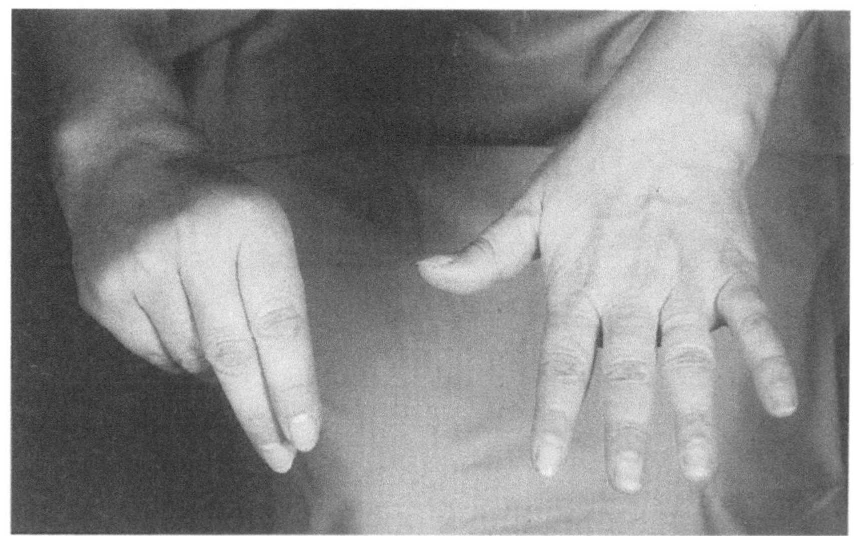

Fig. 7. Posterior interosseous nerve palsy of right hand in rheumatoid arthritis (from [3])

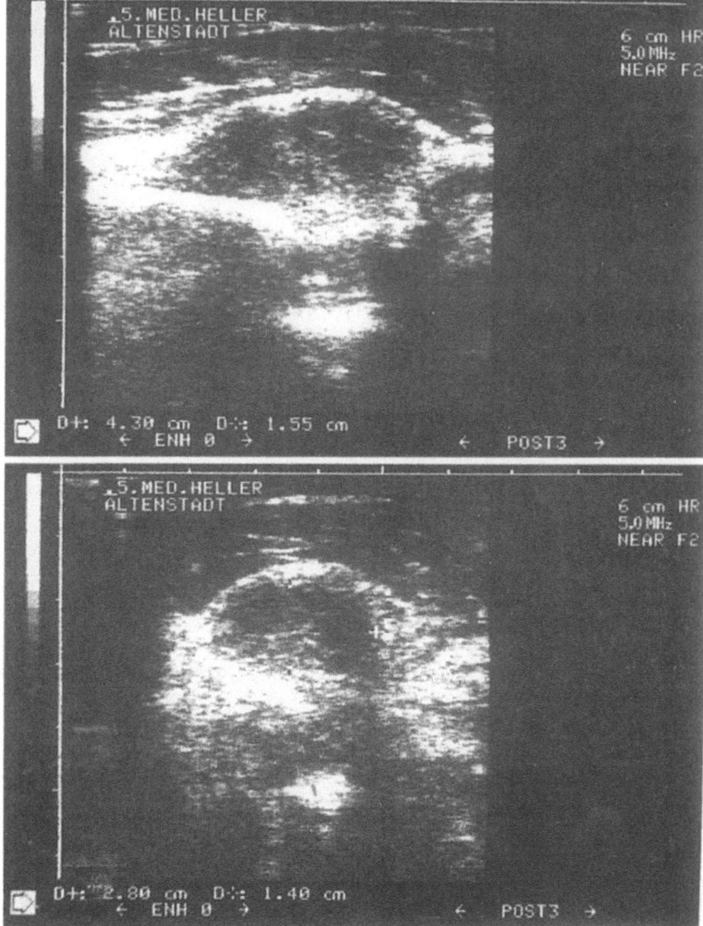

Fig. 8. Sonography of humeroradial joint with anterior compression of radial nerve

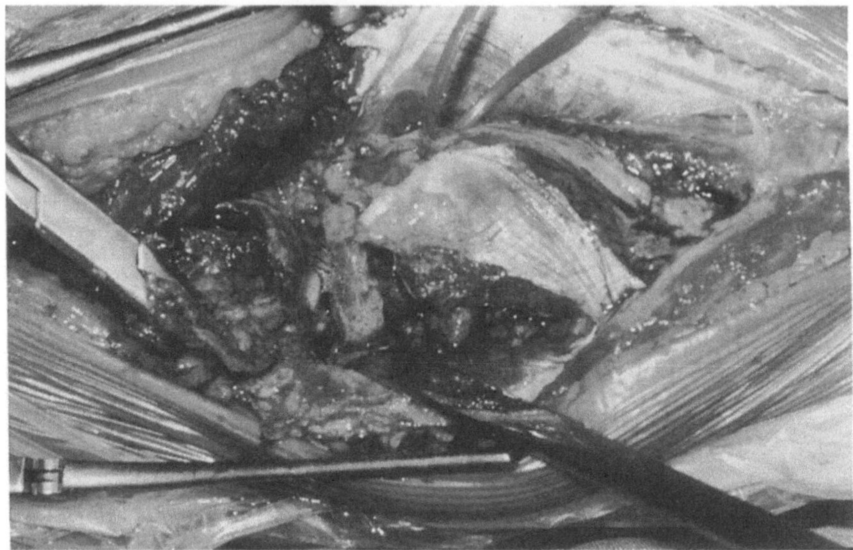

Fig. 9. Synovectomy; radial head resection

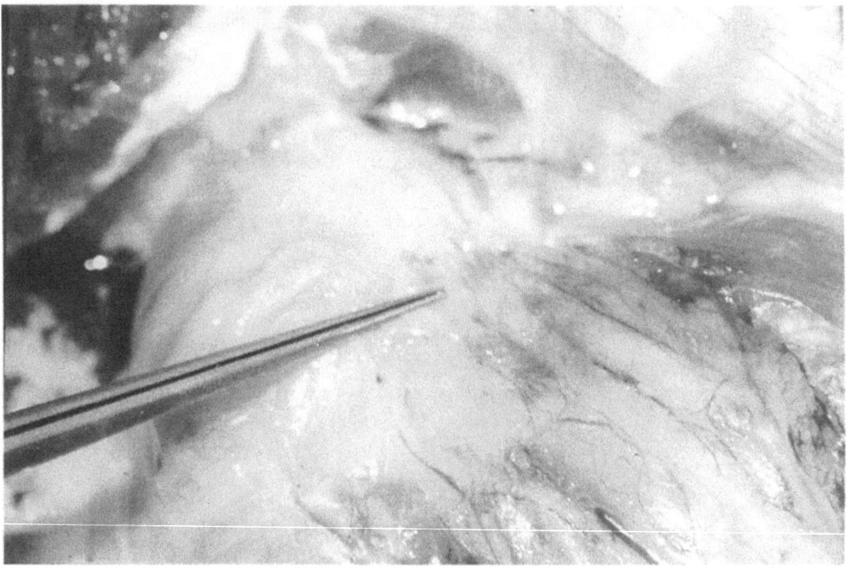

Fig. 10. Decompression of posterior interosseous nerve (magnification)

Surgery of Rheumatoid Elbow Arthritis

The goal of surgery in elbow arthritis should be pain relief and/or restoration of a sufficient range of motion and stability.

Radiosynoviorthesis and Synovectomy (Table 1)

For early stages of the disease, radiosynoviorthesis with rhenium, erbium, yttrium, or dysprosium [9, 21, 28]. is widely used. It is my opinion that this very effective treatment should be reserved for stages 0 and 1 according to Larsen, Dale, and Eek [16]. In late stages, the cartilage thickness decreases, with the potential risk of irradiation of the subchondral bone.

Most authors agree that synovectomy of the elbow gives good results with appreciable pain relief [7, 10, 27, 30]. Synovectomy may be indicated for stages 0–3, although we prefer open synovectomy for stages 2 and 3. A large radial approach by detaching all forearm extensors of the radial side, section of the annular ligament of the radius, and adduction and supination of the forearm according to Banks and Laufmann [1] gives a wide exposure for synovectomy of the whole joint (Figs. 11, 12). Resection of the radial head is avoided whenever possible. Only compressive neuropathy of the ulnar nerve necessitates an ulnar incision for nerve decompression and/or transposition.

For 1 year now my preference for early stages has been a combination of arthroscopic synovectomy and rhenium radiosynoviorthesis 8 weeks later. This treatment has been used for 6 years for knee arthritis in our department and has proved to be very effective.

Arthroplasty (Table 2)

Resection and resection interpositional arthroplasty is a established procedure with acceptable and good results [5, 8, 17].

Table 1. Synovectomy results

Authors	Joints (n)	Follow-up (years)	Good results (%)
Kerschbaumer and Giner [16]	20	4.5	76
Gschwendt and Steiger [10]	40	3	82.5
Ferlic et al. [7]	57	7	77
Tulp and Winia [30]	61	6.5	67

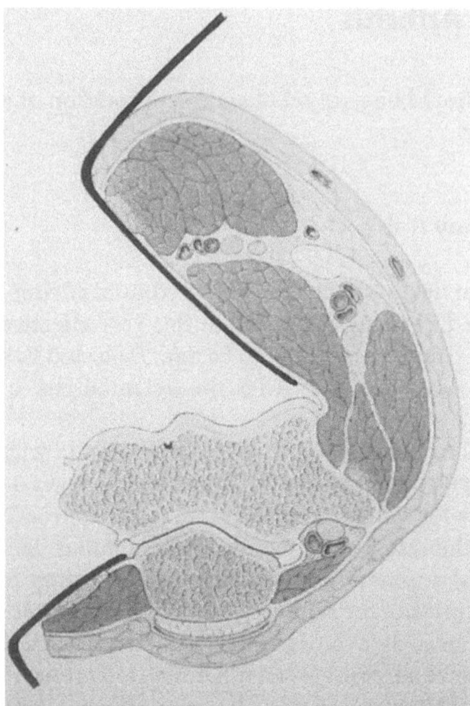

Fig. 11. Large radiodorsal approach for synovectomy

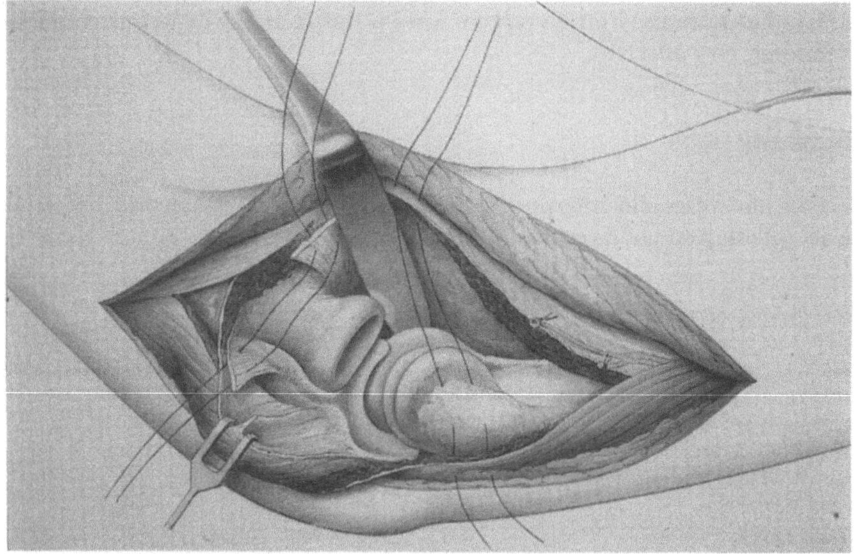

Fig. 12. Detachment and reinsertion of all extensor muscles from humerus (from [2])

Table 2. Total elbow arthroplasty results

Authors	Joints (n)	Follow-up (years)	Good results (%)
Morrey et al. [23]	58	3.8	91
Sjöden and Blomgren [29]	13	5	76
Ewald et al. [6]	202	5.8	91

The indication for this type of surgery is the late stages 4 and 5. The best indication is probably stage 5 with marked pain, acceptable stability, and poor bone stock. The advantage of the resection arthroplasty is durability and an important pain relief. The results in flail elbows are not predictable. In rheumatoid arthritis the techniques described by Haas [11] and Herbert [12] are no longer used. Bone resection should be as minimal as possible; the technique described by Tillmann (this volume) is recommended.

An alternative surgical method for reconstruction of the rheumatoid elbow is total elbow arthroplasty. Early designs of constrained prostheses by Dee, McKee, and Gschwend were not successful because of loosening. With newer semi-constrained prostheses [4, 6, 13, 29] better midterm results have been published, but the complication rate of 15%–40% due to instability, dislocation, or ulnar nerve irritation and infection remains too high.

Conclusion

Destruction, pain, and instability of the rheumatoid elbow may diminish the function of the upper extremity due to a deterioration of the range of motion and/or entrapment neuropathies.

Early treatment by arthroscopic synovectomy and/or radiosynoviorthesis is recommended. For stages 2 and 3, open synovectomy, sometimes in association with nerve decompression, is the treatment of choice. In later stages resection or total elbow arthroplasty is indicated in order to gain a better range of motion and pain relief.

References

1. Banks SV, Laufmann H (1968) An atlas of surgical exposure of the extremities. Saunders, Philadelphia
2. Bauer R, Kerschbaumer F, Poisel S (1987) Operative approaches in orthopedic surgery. Thieme, Stuttgart
3. Bingmann M, Kerschbaumer F (1990) Kompressionssyndrome peripherer Nerven an Ellenbogen und proximalem Unterarm bei chronischer Polyarthritis. Orthop Praxis 26:5–7
4. Dennis DA, Clayton ML, Ferlic DC, Stringer EA, Bramlett KW (1990) Capitello-condylar total elbow arthroplasty for rheumatoid arthritis. J Arthroplasty 5[Suppl]:S83–88

5. Dichson RA, Stein H, Bentley G (1976) Excision arthroplasty of the elbow in rheumatoid disease. J Bone Joint Surg [Br] 58:227–229
6. Ewald FC, Simmons ED Jr, Sullivan JA, Thomas WH, Scott RD, Poss R, Thornhill TS, Sledge CB (1993) Capitellocondylar total elbow replacement in rheumatoid arthritis. J Bone Joint Surg [Am] 75(4):498–507
7. Ferlic DC, Patchett CE, Clayton ML, Freeman AC (1987) Elbow synovectomy in rheumatoid arthritis. Long-term results. Clin Orthop 220:119–125
8. Ferlic D, Clayton M, Parr P. Surgery of the elbow in RA. J Bone Joint Surg [Am] 58:726
9. Gregoir C, Menkes CJ (1991) The rheumatoid elbow: patterns of joint involvement and the outcome of synoviorthesis (published erratum appears in: Ann Chir Main Membr Super 10(6):540, 1991). Ann Chir Main Membr Super 10(3):243–246
10. Gschwend N, Steiger JU (1986) Ellbogengelenk. Orthopäde 15:304–312
11. Haas J (1944) Functional arthroplasty. J Bone Joint Surg Am 26:297
12. Herbert JJ (1958) Traitement des ankyloses du coude dans le rhumatisme
13. Jonsson B, Larsson SE (1990) Elbow arthroplasty in rheumatoid arthritis. Function after 1–2 years in 20 cases. Acta Orthop Scand 61(4):344–347
14. Kerschbaumer F (1988) Orthopade 17
15. Kerschbaumer F (1995) Orthopädische Operationslehre, vol 3. Thieme, Stuttgart
16. Kerschbaumer F, Giner (1986) Operative Therapie am Ellbogen bei cP. In: Des Ellbogen. ML-Velag, Uelzen
17. Kimura C, Vainio K (1976) Arthroplasty of the elbow in rheumatoid arthritis. Arch Orthop Unfall Chir 84:339–348
18. Laine V, Vainio K (1969) Frühsynovectomie bei cP Doc Geigy, Acta Rheumatol S 40
19. Larsen A, Dale K, Eek M (1977) Radiographic evaluation of rheumatoid arthritis and related conditions by standard reference films. Acta Radiol 18(4):481
20. Marmor L, Lawrence JF, Dupois EL (1967) Postereor interosseus nerve palsy due to rheumatoid arthritis. J Bone Joint Surg [Am] 49:319
21. Menkes C, Ingrand J, Paris M (1982) Clinical results with radiosynoviorthesis. In: Kolarz G, Thumb N (eds) Methods of nuclear medical rheumatology. Schattauer, Stuttgart, p 131
22. Millender L, Nalebuff E, Holdworth D (1973) Posterior interosseous nerve syndrome secondary to rheumatoid synovitis. J Bone Joint Surg [Am] 55:753
23. Morrey BF, Adams RA (1992) Semiconstrained arthroplasty for the treatment of rheumatoid arthritis of the elbow. J Bone Joint Surg [Am] 74(4):479–490
24. Nakano K (1975) The entrapment neuropathies of RA. Ortop Chir North Am 6:837
25. Pulkki T, Vainino K (1962) Compression of the ulnar nerve due to rheumatoid arthritis of the elbow. Ann Chir Gynaecol Fenn 51:327
26. Rask M (1979) Anterior interosseous nerve entrapment. Chir Orthop 142:176
27. Raunio P, Pätiälä H (1973) Synovectomie des Ellbogengelenkes. Orthopade 2:28
28. Sledge CB (1984) Intra-artikular radiation synovectomy Clin Orthop 182:37
29. Sjöden G, Blomgren G (1992) The Souter-Strathclyde elbow replacement in rheumatoid arthritis. 13 patients followed for 5 (1–9) years. Acta Orthop Scand 63(3):315–317
30. Tulp NJ, Winia WP (1985) Synovectomy of the elbow in rheumatoid arthritis. Long-term results. J Bone Joint Surg [Br] 71(4):664–666
31. Wörner A (1979) Prozentuale Häufigkeit des Gelenkbefalles bei cP. Dissertation, University of Mainz

The Post-Traumatic Elbow – General Considerations

M. Hansis and S. Arens

Introduction

There are three problems in the follow-up treatment of accidents which can cause the patient and doctor to plan further reconstructive measures at the elbow joint: (1) the post-traumatic reduction of motion, (2) extensive post-traumatic pain, or (3) persisting post-traumatic infection which can not be managed in another way.

Additional objective findings, for example a relevant axial deviation (to be expected up to 50% in children with condylar fractures [10]), extensive defects of the articular surface, or radiologically confirmed, obvious arthrosis (to be expected up to 15%–20% in adults with condylar fractures [10]), certainly represent essential further information. However, from the patients point of view these findings alone do not necessarily make extended operative measures inevitable.

The aim of every extended operative (re)constructive procedure at the elbow joint is the improvement of function (in terms of extension and flexion as well as in terms of supination and pronation), pain relief, stability, and absence of infection. To reach these aims the following techniques are available: (a) open arthrolysis (if necessary with simultaneous removal of periarticular ossifications), (b) resection arthroplasty, (c) endoprothesis, and (d) arthrodesis.

This report will focus on the indication, the expected advantages, and the disadvantages of these four procedures in formerly injured patients.

Other techniques, for example the correction of axis, the removal of pseudarthrosis, or the reestablishing of stability by reconstruction of the coronoid process have their own indications, which are clearly defined and limited. Therefore, in the following report they will not be taken into consideration.

It is necessary to demonstrate how the specific features that are immanent to the above-mentioned operative procedures are superimposed by the formerly injured patients due to completely different considerations and requests: profession, injury of neighbouring joints and, in particular, the effect of getting used to a certain pattern of trauma sequel.

Procedures

Open Arthrolysis

Open arthrolysis (with or without removal of radiologically visible periarticular ossifications) is the most frequently performed intervention of the four above-mentioned procedures. The optimal timing for this operation is approximately 3–6 months after the accident [16], i.e., on the one hand, as soon after the injury as possible and, on the other hand, only when the radiologically confirmed ossifications are smooth and if there is no more irritation of the soft tissue [2, 10, 16]. The indication for the intervention is mainly based on the patient's desire to improve function. In general, a deficit of extension as well as for flexion of at least 40° in either sense is mandatory [10].

The main operative steps are clearing of the olecranon fossa and coronoid fossa, disinsertion of contracted muscles including opening of the ventral capsule, resection of bony edges and chips, mobilization of soft tissue next to the epicondyles, and, far as possible, the removal of implanted foreign material [10, 17] as well as subsequent intensive physiotherapy including application of the continuous passive motion (CPM) machine. Improvement of movement can be expected in approximately 60% of cases [10]. The relative gain of motion is in the range of 15%–65%, depending in particular on the initial situation [1, 12, 13, 17]; improvement of motion can even be confirmed after more than 10 years of follow-up [18]. Preexisting arthrosis impairs the prognosis [17]. For minimal intra-articular changes, arthrolysis can also be done arthroscopically [4].

In addition to the relatively favorable prognosis, the main advantage of open arthrolysis is the fact that, provided there is an uncomplicated course, no additional disadvantages or risks normally have to be taken into account. In contrast to resection arthroplasty, arthrolysis does not regulary lead to loss of stability. Therefore, even in unsuccessful cases (perioperative complications excluded), the preoperative situation can be reestablished after arthrolysis, i.e., the arthrolysis would be unsuccessful, but not associated with an additional disadvantage.

In spite of these relatively favorable conditions, open arthrolysis as a therapeutical measure is only seldom accepted by formerly injured patients. According to our own observations, less then one half of the injured patients taken into consideration consent to this procedure, although it is indicated.

Resection Arthroplasty

Resection arthroplasty of the elbow joint entails resection of the weight-bearing joint surfaces and interposition of strips from the fascia. It is indicated for painful and extensive stiffness of the elbow joint, i.e., for severe post-traumatic arthrosis. The leading clinical signs can be extensive limitation of flexion (if the hand cannot reach the mouth and neck), extensive limitation of extension or rotational movement of the forearm (which can be very inconvenient in everyday life), or unbearable pain. A precondition for resection arthroplasty is a joint free of any irritation with good muscle splinting, as only then can the loss of passive stability be partially compensated. The main disadvantage of resection arthroplasty is the "inevitable reciprocal relation between stability and mobility," which makes it difficult to predict the results [3]. The indication is most convincing if there is an infection which cannot be managed otherwise and where compression arthrodesis is the only altenative [9].

Endoprothesis

Total endoprothedic replacement of the elbow joint for post-traumatic conditions is only seldomly indicated (Ruth [15], only two out of 41 patients). This is because of the relatively high rates of early complications [7, 8] and not always satisfactory long-term stability [3, 7]. The fact that, after an average observation period of approximately 5 years, 45% bad results can be expected induced Morrey [7] to advise against the treatment of formerly injured patients with endoprothesis of the elbow joint. A more accepted indication is the isolated replacement of the radial head [6, 14], which leads to good results in about two thirds of cases. These can still be confirmed after an observation period of more than 10 years [5].

Arthrodesis

Arthrodesis of the elbow joint leads without doubt to very good stability and generally to considerable pain reduction or even painlessness. However, the total loss of flexion and extension as well as the loss of rotational movement of the forearm has to be considered as an extremely serious disadvantage. Cinemato-graphic studies in which the condition of arthrodesis was simulated using an immobilizing brace demonstrated that, even with full function of the equilateral shoulder and wrist joint, the suspended function of the elbow joint after arthrodesis cannot be compensated at all [11]. Therefore, the indication for arthrodesis should be assessed even more cautiously than for the other three measures (especially in the case of infection which cannot be managed otherwise [9] or in the case of an arthrotic, completely destroyed, wobbling, stiff, and very painful joint [16]). Furthermore, in exceptional cases arthrodesis can be indicated in the case of muscular paralysis to reestablish a certain passive stability [10].

Expectations Concerning the Operative Intervention and Remarks on the Choice of Procedure

Coinjury of Other Joints

Excellent cooperation on the part of the patient, local tissue conditions without any irritation, and good function of the equilateral shoulder and wrist joint are preconditions for open arthrolysis of the elbow joint. The patient has to be able to concentrate entirely on the postoperative treatment after this intervention. Therefore, the performance of other demanding operative procedures in other areas does not appear to be advisable.

For resection arthroplasty sufficient muscular splinting or muscular hold of the joint is absolutely necessary. The same is true for the implantation of an endoprothesis. In this case, the patient should also be free of any source of bacterial dissemination. For both interventions it is important that the traumatized patient does not depend on the ability to support an extensive passive load on the arm, as for example in the case of a fracture that has not yet united or after amputation in the area of the lower extremities. For paraplegic patients, it must be considered very carefully whether the expected increase in motion will really be an advantage or whether the loss of stability after resection arthroplasty and/or the limited tolerance to longer weight-bearing are not more disadvantageous. Furthermore, resection arthroplasty and implantation of an endoprothesis can be restricted by post-traumatic damage of local soft tissue.

An absolutely necessary requirement for arthrodesis is an excellent range of movement of the equilateral shoulder and wrist joint.

Profession

An important factor in the choice of the procedure is based on the profession and the professional plans of the formerly injured patient.

In the case of severe arthrotic destruction of the elbow joint after percondylar fracture of the humerus associated with painful wobbling and stiffness, an injured 35-year-old farmer who has to support the whole family would probably prefer arthrodesis, because freedom from pain and stability are far more important in his situation than improved range of movement. In contrast, a graphic artist with comparable initial findings would probably prefer resection arthroplasty or even endoprothesis; the gradual gain of motion will be so important for him that he will presumably accept either a certain primary loss of stability (in the case of resection arthroplasty) or limited long-term stability (in the case of endoprothesis). Finally, a 35-year-old housewife who has to care for three small children and run the household will presumably initially decide against any operative treatment and try to cope with the immediate result of treatment. Being away from home due to several weeks of treatment and the uncertainities connected with all the available therapeutical measures will motivate this decision.

Time Course

The dynamics of the course of illness is very important for formerly injured patients in their decision for or against a certain follow-up treatment (as well as in the choice between the four above-mentioned interventions at the elbow).

Patients with rheumatoid arthritis suffer from a progressive illness which attacks and increasingly destroys more or less all the joints. They suffer from an illness characterized by continuous progression. The central objective of every therapeutical measure is to halt this progression as far as possible and, at the same time, to regain satisfying residual function of the joint. For rheumatoid patients, therefore, what counts is the chance to prevent further, even worse deterioration (in terms of pain, stability, or movement), e.g., by undergoing arthroplasty. The situation is similar for patients suffering from nonmanageable infection.

The chronological course of the illness is reversed in traumatic patients. After inital quite favorable conditions (in terms of pain and movement), during the immediate postoperative treatment there is a constant improvement to start with. After a certain time, injured patients will achieve a steady state (concerning pain and movement). Once they and their doctor realize that they have reached this steady state, they generally start to reconsider whether at least one of the three main qualities (pain, movement, and stability) can be effectively improved by operative measures without causing a deterioration in one of the other qualities. For the injured patient, the goal is not to stop a constant downward progression, but to take the chance to improve a moderate treatment result into a somewhat better one.

As always for comparable considerations in general, in operative procedures at the elbow joint the demands are quite high, as far as the benefit to be expected, the risks associated with the treatment, and the suspected disadvantages related to the treatment are concerned. Patients will carefully consider the therapeutic measures available with regard to their personal situation under three main aspects, namely personal adaptation to the condition, the probability of improvement, and especially the probability of deterioration.

Thus it is understandable why, for example, endoprothesis of the elbow joint or resection arthroplasty are unlikely to be accepted by the patient. In terms of adaptation, hardly any patient will be prepared to accept a disadvantage in the hope (but not certainty) of gaining an advantage. It becomes understandable why, of the described procedures, only open arthrolysis is performed routinely: for this procedure the success of treatment is uncertain, but the injured patients generally (with the exception of manifest complications) do not have to take predictable disadvantages into account.

Only for chronic post-traumatic infection is the situation different. Here, formerly traumatized patients are in a difficult situation (similar to patients suffering from progressive rheumatoid arthritis): at a certain stage of the infection, they basically have no other option than to agree to arthrodesis or resection arthroplasty.

Conclusion

In addition to their advantages, resection arthroplasty, arthrodesis, endoprothesis, and open arthrolysis each have independant and typical disadvantages. Most of all, limited tolerance to longer weight-bearing in the case of endoprothesis and the immediate loss of stability caused by resection arthroplasty are, with good reason, considered to be very serious by patients who work (and therefore by the majority of formerly injured patients). The indication for endoprothesis, resection arthroplasty, arthrodesis, or open arthrolysis in formerly injured patients must therefore be considered much less under the aspect of the objective initial findings and more in terms of the benefit to be expectetd, the likely disadvantages, and, in particular, with regards to the age and profession of the patient. For the trauma patient, at the time of decision for one of the above-mentioned steps in the follow-up treatment concept, adaptation is of primary importance: injured patients reach an individual steady state in terms of movement, stability, and pain to which they adapt according to the circumstances. With the exception of those suffering from chronic infection, patients are therefore not willing to merely prevent continous deterioration, but will wish to transform a moderate result into a better one. For this reason, certain advantages and disadvantages of the proposed operation will be measured first and foremost in terms of the level of adaptation.

If open arthrolysis, resection arthroplasty, arthrodesis, or endoprothesis is to be performed in formerly injured patients, the treating doctor first has to estimate at an early post-traumatic stage the further course, taking two main considerations into account. He or she has to estimate when and at what level the steady state phase in terms of movement and low-grade pain will be reached and by which procedure and with what probability a better result could be achieved. The earlier this can be estimated and the more certain it is, the earlier the treating doctor will be able to take measures to prevent the traumatized patient from entering the phase of adaptation to the steady state and the more convincingly and certainly he or she will probably be able to guide the patient to an even better overall result. For this the most essential precondition is the ability to foresee in as exact a way as possible the effect of the proposed operative treatment measures.

References

1. Breitfuß H, Muhr G, Neumann K, Neumann C, Rehn J (1991) Die Arthrolyse posttraumatischer Ellbogensteifen Unfallchirurg 94:33–39
2. Garland DE, Hanscom DA, Keenan MA, Smith C, Muhr T (1985) Resection of heterotopic ossification in the adult with head trauma. J Bone Joint Surg 67A:1261–1269
3. Gschwend N (1986) Degenerative Erkrankungen der oberen Extremität. Z Orthop 124:408–417
4. Jerosch H, Castro WHM (1992) Arthroskopie des Ellbogengelenkes. Unfallchirurg 95:405–411
5. Lies A, Josten C, Visel C, Ekkernkamp A (1993) Spärtergebnisse nach dem Einbau von Radiusköpfchenprothesen. 57th Annual Meeting of the DGU (Berlin) 1993 (lecture)
6. Mittelmeier T, Hertlein H, Schümann M, Lob G (1993) Primäre und früh-sekundäre Indikation zu endoprothetischen Radiusköpfchenersatz. 57th Annual Meeting of the DGU (Berlin) 1993 (lecture)
7. Morrey BF, Bryan RS (1987) Revision total elbow arthroplasty. J Bone Joint Surg 69A:523–532
8. Morrey BF, Adams RA (1992) Semiconstrained arthroplasty for the treatment of rheumatoid arthritis of the elbow. J Bone Joint Surg 74A:479–490
9. Muhr G, Kayser M (1988) Die infizierte Ellbogengelenkfraktur. Orthopade 17:279–286
10. Mutschler W, Burri C, Rübenacker S (1990) Rekonstruktive Chirurgie fehlverheilter Ellbogengelenkbrüche. Orthopade 19:324–331

11. O'Neill OR, Morrey BF, Tanaka S, A, KN (1992) Compensatory motion in the upper extremity after elbow arthrodesis. Orthop Relat Res 281:89–96
12. Neumann K, Breitfuss H, Muhr G (1993) Remobilisierende Operationen nach posttraumatischen Ellenbogengelenks-einsteifungen – Wann und wie? 57th Annual Meeting of the DGU (Berlin) 1993 (lecture)
13. Rudolph H, Dölle H, Mommsen U, Jungbluth KH (1976) Indikation und Ergebnisse der Osteosynthese von Trümmerbrüchen in Ellenbogen-gelenksbereich besonders bei älteren Patienten. H Unfallheilk 126:370–372
14. Rüter A (1981) Der veraltete Speichenköpfchenbruch – operative Behandlungsmöglichkeiten. Unfallmedizinische Tagungen der Landesverbände der Gewerblichen. Berufsgenossenschaften 46:85–95
15. Ruth JT, Wilde AJ (1992) Capitellocondylar total elbow replacement. A long-term follow-up study. J Bone Joint Surg 74A:95–100
16. Schmit-Neuerburg KP, Assenmacher S (1986) Prinzipien von Diagnostik, Indikationsstellung und Therapiekonzepten Unfallmedizinische Tagungen der Landesverbände der Gewerblichen. Berufsgenossenschaften 70:171–181
17. Urbaniak JR, Hansen PE, Beissinger SF, Aitken MS (1985) Correction of post-traumatic flexion contracture of the elbow by anterior capsulotomy. J Bone Joint Surg 67A:1160–1165
18. Wirth CJ (1991) Spätergebnisse nach Arthrolyse und Arthroplastik des Ellenbogengelenkes. H Unfallheilkd 220:57–58

Anatomy, Biomechanics, and Kinematics of Total Elbow Replacement

M.P. Figgie

Anatomy

Elbow Joint

The elbow joint consists of the articulations of the distal humerus, proximal ulna, and proximal radius. The distal humerus has two condyles: the trochlea on the medial aspect and the capitellum on the lateral aspect. The trochlea articulates with the proximal ulna, whereas the capitellum articulates with the proximal radius. The ulnohumeral articulation acts as a hinged joint (ginglymus) with degrees of freedom in flexion and extension. However, An et al. showed that the elbow is not a true hinge, as there is varus and valgus laxity of 3°–4° [27]. The radiohumeral joint and the proximal radioulnar joint allow axial rotation with pronation and supination and thus represent a trochoid joint. Based upon these two articulations, the elbow is a trochoginglymoid joint [36].

The trochlea itself is bicondylar and saddle shaped, with an asymmetric joint surface between the medial and lateral condyles. Hyaline cartilage covers it in an arc that varies from 300° to 330° [14, 35, 37].

The capitellum is spheroidal, articulating with the concave aspects of the proximal radius [37]. The depression of the radial head is covered by hyaline cartilage as well as the 240° arc of circumference that articulates with the ulna, allowing approximately 180° of pronation and supination.

The proximal ulna consists of the olecranon, the site of the attachment for the triceps tendon. The greater sigmoid notch, which articulates with the trochlea at the humerus, is incompletely covered with hyaline cartilage [37]. The anterior aspect of the sigmoid notch consists of the coronoid process. The insertion of the brachialis muscle is distal to the coronoid tip and does not attach to the tip directly. Along the lateral aspect of the proximal ulna, the lesser semilunar notch articulates with the large circumferential margin of the proximal radius. The radius is stabilized by the annular ligament, which circumscribes the neck of the radius.

The extra-articular landmarks of the elbow include the medial and lateral epicondyles of the distal humerus. The medial epicondyle is more proximal and is the site of attachment of the ulnar collateral ligament and the flexor and pronator musculature of the forearm. The lateral epicondyle is the site of attachment of the lateral collateral ligament and the mobile wad of three muscles: the brachioradialis muscle, the long radial extensor muscle of the wrist, and the short radial extensor muscle of the wrist. The posterior aspect of the lateral epicondyle is the origin of the anconeus muscle. The ulnar nerve lies in a sulcus of the cubital tunnel distal to the medial epicondyle. The distal humerus has three recesses or sulci, which allow for a greater range of motion of the elbow. The coronoid fossa accommodates the coronoid process, whereas the radial fossa, which is above the surface of the capitellum, accommodates the radial head with elbow flexion. The olecranon fossa, which is posterior, accommodates the tip of the olecranon in full extension. The coronoid and olecranon fossae are supported by the medial and lateral supracondylar ridges of the distal humerus. The supracondylar ridges or pillars provide support to most designs of semiconstrained total elbow replacements. In addition, they are important structures in the open reduction and internal fixation of distal humeral fractures. The lateral supracondylar column is larger with a flat posterior surface, whereas the medial supracondylar pillar is smaller.

The orientation of the elbow joint articulation with the shafts of the humerus and ulna must be appreciated in order to properly restore the anatomic relationships with total elbow replacement. The trochlea and capitellum are angulated at 30° anterior to the long axis of the humerus (Fig. 1). The center of the rotation of

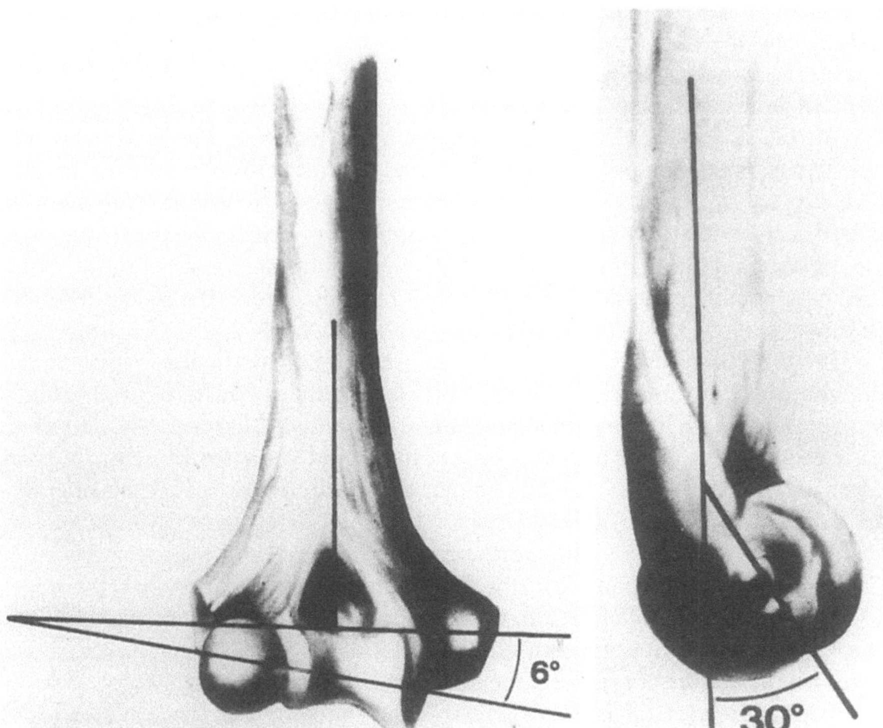

Fig. 1. The center of rotation is angulated anteriorly with regard to the humeral shaft

Fig. 2. The distal humerus has a 4°–6° valgus angulation with regard to the shaft

the articulation is approximately 6°–8° of valgus orientation to the long axis of the humerus [17]. In addition, the axis is internally rotated to 5°–7° from the line bisecting the epicondyles [18] (Fig. 2).

There is a 15° angle of the neck of the radius with respect to the long axis of the radius [2] and a 4° valgus angulation of the olecranon with respect to the shaft of the ulna [15].

The carrying angle of the elbow is provided by the valgus angle of the humeral articulation with the long axis of the humerus and the valgus angle of the sigmoid notch with the long axis of the ulna. This angle is the relationship of the long axis of the forearm to the long axis of the humerus with the arm extended. In a patient with multiple joint disease, this angle allows the patient to reach the face more easily than if the axis of the forearm and humerus were parallel.

Soft Tissues

The elbow is supported by the medial and lateral collateral ligament complexes. The medial collateral ligament is more discrete, consisting of three bundles: anterior, posterior, and transverse. The anterior portion extends from the medial epicondyle to the sublimis tubercle of the proximal ulna [21, 32]. The posterior portion is well defined only at 90° of flexion and, like the transverse ligament, provides little stability. The tension of the anterior portion of the medial collateral ligament varies with flexion and extension.

The lateral collateral ligament complex is less discrete. The radial collateral ligament originates from the lateral epicondyle and terminates in the annular ligament [14, 24]. The radial collateral ligament appears to be taut throughout the normal range of flexion and extension. The accessory lateral collateral ligament, by comparison, apparently functions only when varus stress is applied to the elbow. The lateral ulnar collateral ligament is a major stabilizer resisting rotary instability [26].

The musculature is described only as it applies to total elbow replacements. The important secondary stabilizers of the elbow joint are the flexor and extensor masses; they attach at the medial and lateral epicondyles, respectively. The flexor mass includes the flexor pronator group: the round pronator muscle, the radial flexor muscle of the wrist, the long palmar muscle, and the ulnar flexor muscle of the wrist. The extensor muscles attaching at the lateral epicondyle include the brachioradialis muscle and the short and long radial extensor muscles of the wrist. The common extensor muscle of the fingers also originates at the anterior aspect of the lateral epicondyle. One head of the ulnar extensor muscle of the wrist originates from the common extensor group. The anconeus muscle, which aids in elbow extension, originates from the posterior aspect of the lateral epicondyle and inserts into the surface of the proximal ulna. The supinator muscle also has an origin on the lateral epicondyle and inserts along the proximal aspect of the ulna along the crista supinatoris.

The major extensor of the elbow is the triceps muscle of the arm. It inserts into the olecranon through a large triceps tendon. Electromyographic studies have indicated that the major flexor of the elbow is the brachialis muscle, inserting at the base of the coronoid process. Although the biceps muscle of the arm aids in forearm flexion, it also acts as a supinator of the forearm [41].

Biomechanics

The normal elbow has an arc of 160° of flexion from full extension, 80° of pronation, and 85° of supination [23]. However, most activities of daily living can be performed with an arc of flexion from 30° to 130°, with a 100° arc of rotation divided equally between pronation and supination [20]. The range of motion of the elbow is thought to be limited by the geometry of the joint surfaces and impingement of the bone on surrounding capsule and muscle. However, the 30° anterior angulation of the distal humerus combined with the coronoid and olecranon fossae help increase the elbow's range of motion [14]. The primary functions of the elbow include positioning the hand in space, providing a stable axis for the forearm as a lever, and functioning as a weight-bearing joint. This last function is of help to patients who use assistive devices for walking, such as crutches and canes [11].

Although the location of the center of rotation of the elbow has been the subject of numerous investigations, no consensus has been reached on the matter. Youm and colleagues concluded that the axis of rotation does not change with flexion and extension [41]. Morrey and Chao [20] have suggested that the instant centers vary and that the elbow is not a true hinge joint, but that deviations from the center of rotation are minimal through most of the arc of motion, occurring mainly at the extremes of motion. Thus, the axis of rotation could be assumed to be a single joint at the center of the circle formed by the trochlear sulcus and capitellum [18].

Elbow joint reaction forces of up to two to three times body weight can be generated with normal activities of daily living [23]. Torzilli demonstrated that the biceps muscle must generate up to 38 times the static force applied to the extended elbow because of the short moment arm of the muscular attachment with relationship to the relatively long moment arm of the applied force [38]. Dynamic loading, occurring when one lifts an object, rises from a seated position with the aid of the arm, or uses an assistive device to walk, may generate peaks of more than six times the body weight. For the purposes of implant design, therefore, the elbow must be considered a weight-bearing joint.

Walker [40], Hui and associates [9], and Pearson and associates [29] determined that the largest joint reaction forces were directed in a posterior plane at the distal humerus. The forces may result in posterior shifting of a prosthetic humeral component with anterior rotation and stem pressure along the anterior humeral cortex.

Rotational stresses along the total elbow replacement may also be high, especially in the patient with a stiff shoulder. In this patient, the transmission of loads to the bone – cement interface of the elbow replacement increase during attempts to internally and externally rotate the arm.

Stability of the elbow joint is provided by joint surface congruity, static soft tissue stabilization, including that of the medial and lateral collateral ligaments, and dynamic stabilization, including that of the flexor and extensor muscle masses attaching at the epicondyles. The ulnohumeral joint is quite congruous, accounting for almost 50% of its stability. The anterior capsule provides 70% of soft tissue restraint to distraction in extension, and the medial collateral ligament assumes this function at 90° of flexion. In extension, varus stress is resisted equally by the joint articulation and the soft tissues, including the lateral collateral ligament and capsule. In flexion, the joint congruity provides 75% of the resistance to varus stress [22].

Resistance to valgus stress in extension is divided equally between the medial collateral ligament and the joint congruency in concert with the capsule. Valgus stress with the elbow flexed is primarily stabilized by the medial collateral ligament. A secondary stabilizer is joint congruency. Because the origin of the medial collateral ligament is not at the center of rotation, the anterior portion of the ligament is taut during extension and flexion, and the posterior portion is taut only during flexion [22, 28, 32]. The lateral ligament complex, with its origin at the center of rotation, is taut during flexion and extension. Most activities of daily living are performed with the elbow flexed and result in valgus stress along the elbow. Thus, the medial collateral ligament, providing over 50% of the stability for the joint, is extremely important to function.

Removal of the radial head places further demands on the medial collateral ligament as joint congruency is lost, and valgus stress must be resisted almost entirely by the medial collateral ligament. Approximately 60% of the stress is shared by the radiohumeral articulation with the elbow extended and axially loaded [8]. In addition, with the elbow flexed, tensile forces may reach twice the body weight in the medial collateral ligament, whereas compressive forces on the radial head may reach up to three times the body weight [1]. Excision of the radial head may result in greater stress in the medial collateral ligament of up to nine times the body weight.

Kinematics of Total Elbow Replacement

Current designs of total elbow replacement differ in their fixation, articulation, and amount of constraint. The early designs of total elbow replacement were fixed hinges including the Dee and the Gschwend-Scheier-Bähler (GSB) I designs. However, these implants often failed rapidly due to the increased stresses at the bone – cement interface secondary to the highly constrained articulation. In addition, metal-on-metal wear may have contributed to loosening [6]. This led to the design of semiconstrained and nonconstrained prostheses. Nonconstrained prostheses, which are dependent upon soft tissues for stability, theoretically have lower loosening rates, but higher dislocation rates. The semiconstrained implants have lower dislocation rates, but may have higher loosening rates. In addition, polyethylene wear may be problematic in either type of implant over long periods of use.

Hinged Devices

Most hinged devices are no longer utilized. The only recent report on a hinged device involves the Stanmore total elbow replacement [13]. This long-stemmed device is completely constrained and is available in right and left implants. The joint is angulated with relation to the stem of the implant, and this recreates the carrying angle. The constraint of the implant results in high stresses being transferred to the bone–cement interface.

Semiconstrained Implants

There have been numerous semiconstrained implants including the original Pritchard-Walker, the Pritchard-Walker Mark II, the GSB, the Volz, the three generations of the Coonrad elbow, the triaxial and Osteonics implants. Semiconstrained implants fall into two major categories: the snap-fit devices and the linked components. They are stemmed implants which usually require more bone resection. In addition, since the normal trochlea is offset medially from the stem of the implant, the semiconstrained devices usually move the center of rotation laterally. In this way, the joint's articulation becomes balanced by the flexor and extensor masses of the epicondyles due to the equal offsets from the center of the articulation. Since the medial collateral ligament is elevated with this procedure, the joint center can be shifted laterally and the ligaments can heal in the elongated position.

The early semiconstrained devices allowed little rotation and varus – valgus motion, with the exception of the triaxial implant, which was a sloppy hinge articulation. Most current devices allow for varus, valgus and rotational motion.

Snap-Fit Articulation

There were two implants with snap-fit articulations. These included the triaxial (Fig. 3), and the Volz elbow. The Volz elbow offset the trochlear replacement to its normal medial alignment and allowed for replacement of the radial head. However, there was a high percentage of recurrent dislocations due to wear of the bushing, and this implant is no longer utilized. The triaxial implant was modeled after the original Pritchard-Walker implant and originally had an axle [10]. The articulation was changed to a snap fit and it allowed 10°–12° of motion in the varus–valgus direction and 4°–6° of rotational motion. The elbow also had an appropriate anterior bow, which allowed anatomic reconstruction of the center of rotation. However, dislocations have also occurred with the triaxial implant due to

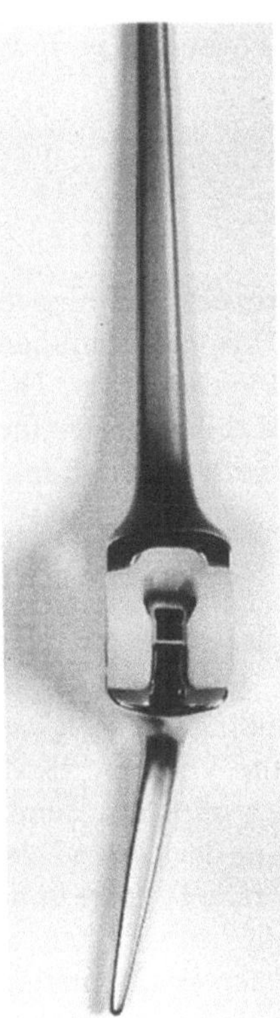

Fig. 3. The triaxial is a snap-fit design with 8°–10° degrees of laxity

polyethylene wear, and a third-generation design includes a linked articulation to prevent this. The Norway elbow is a non-constrained articulation with a spool-type trochlear design with an optional locking ring. This allows for rotational laxity, but, again, the concern is long-term instability secondary to polyethylene wear. The polyethylene spool is at higher risk for wear due to the convex surface of the polyethylene, as polyethylene does not wear as well in a convex shape.

Linked Devices

The early generations of semiconstrained devices are no longer available, including the Mayo, Schlein, Pritchard Mark I, and Coonrad I and II elbows. The Pritchard Mark I device had an all-polyethylene humeral component, which had a high incidence of fracture [10] (Fig. 4). This was changed to a metal humeral component with a polyethylene bushing and an axle. However, it was still fairly constrained and at long-term follow-up failure of the bushings and linkage has occurred.

The GSB implant was redesigned to allow for motion at the bushing of the ulna (Fig. 5). The kinematics of the joint act as a hinge with rotation and varus–valgus laxity due to the ulnar high-density polyethylene bushing [7].

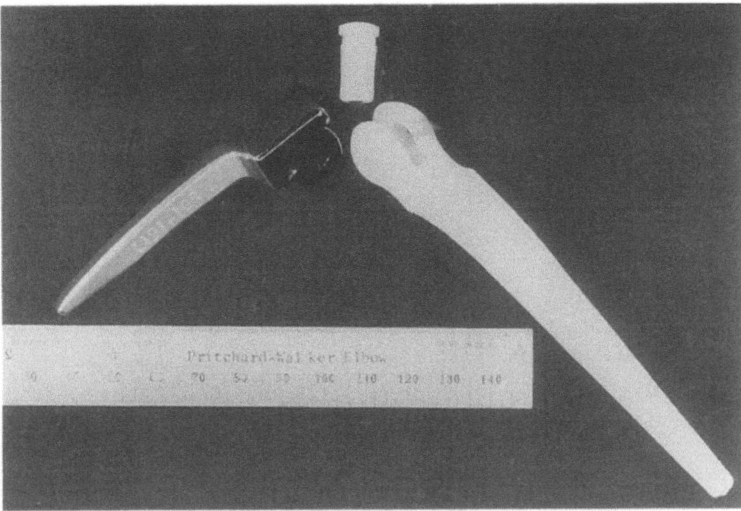

Fig. 4. The Pritchard-Walker Mark I prosthesis had an all-polyethylene humeral component which was prone to fracture

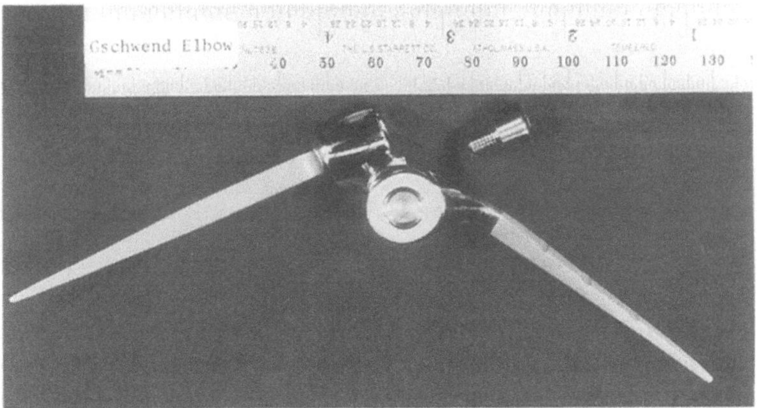

Fig. 5. The Gschwend-Scheier-Bäher (GSB-III) elbow has motion within the ulnar component with a polyethlene bearing

The Coonrad I design was first utilized in 1971 and was a rigid hinged device (Fig. 6). It was modified in 1978 to allow 8° of varus – valgus motion and 8° of axial rotation. In 1981, an anterior flange was added to the distal humeral component to help with rotational stability and help prevent posterior migration [25].

The Osteonics implant, which was based upon the triaxial design, is a linked semiconstrained device which allows for 8° of varus – valgus and rotational motion [5] (Fig. 7). The bearing surface is on a concave polyethylene bushing with convex condyles that articulate only in extremes of motion. The axle is not loaded except with distraction forces.

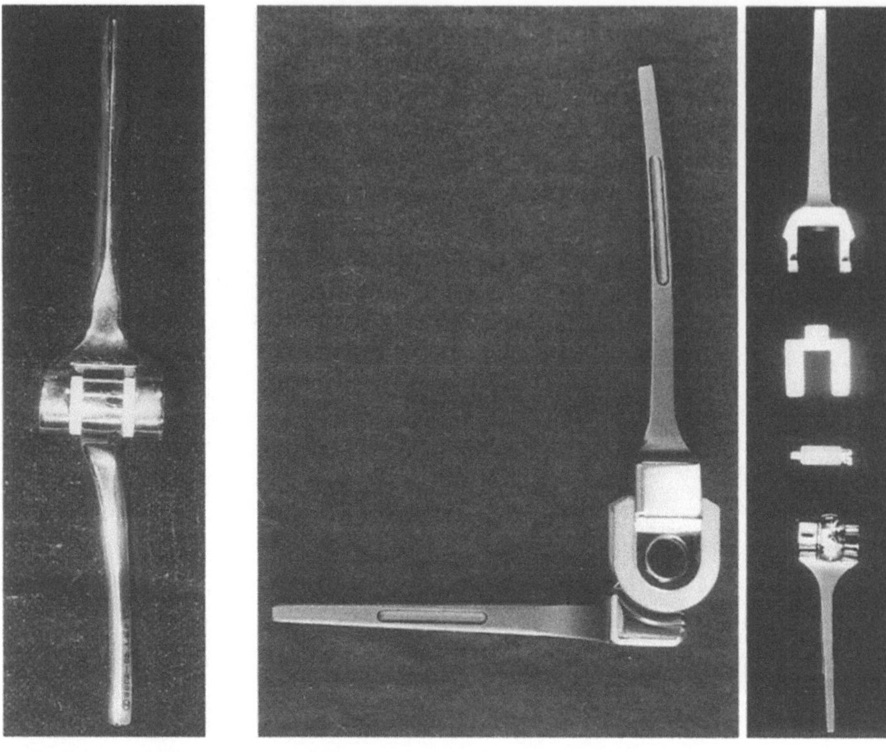

Fig. 6. The original Coonrad implant was hinged. The type II design had more laxity, and the type III has an anterior flange

Fig. 7. a The Osteonics component is semiconstrained with a linked axle which is not load bearing. b The polyethylene is centrally loaded and the condyles take load at extremes of motion

O'Driscoll et al. evaluated the kinematics of the Coonrad III elbow and compared it to the natural elbow [27]. They found that there were 2.7° (±1.5°) of varus and valgus motion in the natural elbow with functional activities. With the total elbow implanted, this increased to 3.8° (±1.4°). Even in the loaded condition, the normal motion of the natural elbow was 6.9° (±3.7°) of valgus and the measurements were 10.8° (±1.8°) with the prosthesis implanted. This study revealed that the modified Coonrad prosthesis behaved as a semiconstrained joint. The functional laxity was less than the actual structural laxity of the implant and thus allowed the soft tissues to resist stress.

Nonconstrained Implants

Nonconstrained implants are dependent upon the static and dynamic soft tissue forces to stabilize the implant. These include the medial and lateral ligament complexes and the dynamic action of the muscles. While most nonconstrained implants employ polyethylene on the concave ulna, some have polyethylene humeral components with convex surfaces, which may result in greater wear. In addition, numerous implants are surface replacements of the distal humerus and do not have stems. Their insertion requires removal of subchondral bone, and the soft distal humeral cancellous bone often fails due to the posterior vector force applied to the humerus. This results in subsidence of the humerus with posterior migration. Both the Kudo and Imperial College and the London Hospital (ICLH) prostheses have been modified to include a stem to help prevent this migration [17, 31]. With the stemmed prostheses, the trochlea must be anatomically restored to provide appropriate soft tissue balance with the medial collateral ligament. In addition, the lateral collateral ligament complex must be accurately restored to prevent translocation and dislocation. The use of radial head replacements has been variable due to difficulty in attempting to balance three joints. However, in nonconstrained implants, the radial head replacement may provide added stability to valgus stress.

Current designs of nonconstrained implants include the capitellocondylar, the Kudo, Souter, Wadsworth, ICLH, Liverpool, Lowe, Norway and Pritchard implants. Each of these differs in their shape and articulation. There are three basic types of articulations: cylindrical, saddle shaped, and bicondylar.

The ICLH implant has a concave, all-polyethylene ulna with a cylindrically shaped distal humerus [31]. The ulna component originally was implanted without a stem. The matching ulna and humeral radii allow for flexion and extension and medial and lateral sliding to allow soft tissue balancing. However, with varus and valgus stress or axial rotation liftoff occurs, causing edge loading on the polyethylene.

The original design of the Kudo prosthesis also had a cylindrical distal humerus with a high-density polyethylene ulnar component [16, 17]. The ulna had a short stem with an articular surface that conformed to the humerus. This was then modified (type II) to a saddle-shaped humeral component. The articulating surface of the ulna had a larger radius of curvature than the humeral component, which allowed for a slight degree of varus and valgus angulation and axial rotation. In 1983, a stem was added to the humeral component to prevent subsidence and posterior migration of the humerus.

There are several nonconstrained elbow replacements which are saddle shaped in nature. These include the Wadsworth, Liverpool, Lowe, and Souter. Both the Lowe and Wadsworth prostheses have all polyethylene humeral components, which again may present problems with higher amounts of wear due to the convex shape [19, 39]. The humeral component of the Wadsworth prosthesis has a concave surface in the coronal plane and a convex surface in the sagittal plane [39]. The ulnar component is made of alivium with a matching articulation and an ulnar stem. The prosthesis does allow for varus and valgus motion; however, axial rotation results in edge loading and liftoff.

The original Lowe prosthesis did not have stems on either the titanium ulnar component or the polyethylene humeral component [19]. A stemmed polyethylene component was later designed for the humerus and a stemmed ulnar component. The articulation is saddle shaped with a distinct central ridge, which may cause high stress concentration. Its articulation does allow for varus and valgus motion, but axial rotation is restricted. In addition, the stems are straight and the trochlea is translocated laterally with insertion. The all-polyethylene humeral component, similar to the original Pritchard-Walker Mark I prosthesis, may be prone to fracture.

The Liverpool prosthesis also had a saddle-shaped distal humerus configuration with stemless ulnar and humeral components [33]. Stems were later added to both components. The carrying angle in the stemless prosthesis is reproduced with the method of surgery. In the stemmed components, the alignment is fixed and the center is moved laterally. In addition, a great deal of bone must be removed to insert the stemmed distal humeral component. The polyethylene ulnar component is not conforming, and the mismatch allows for varus and valgus stress and some axial rotation.

The Souter prosthesis has a saddle-shaped distal humerus with a stirrup for insertion [34]. The all-polyethylene ulnar component has a matching articulation and a high coronoid process. It allows for varus and valgus motion, but axial rotation is restricted. The implant is designed to recreate the carrying angle with 8° of valgus angulation with extension and 6° of varus with flexion.

The capitellocondylar (Fig. 8) and Pritchard systems both have condylar-shaped distal humeri which resemble the trochlea and capitellum of the natural elbow [3, 30]. Both prostheses can be inserted with a radial head replacement. The trochlea is offset from the stem, which allows soft tissue tensioning. The polyethylene ulna has a surface wihch matches the humerus and allows for some varus and valgus angulation and rotational laxity due to the eccentric tracking of

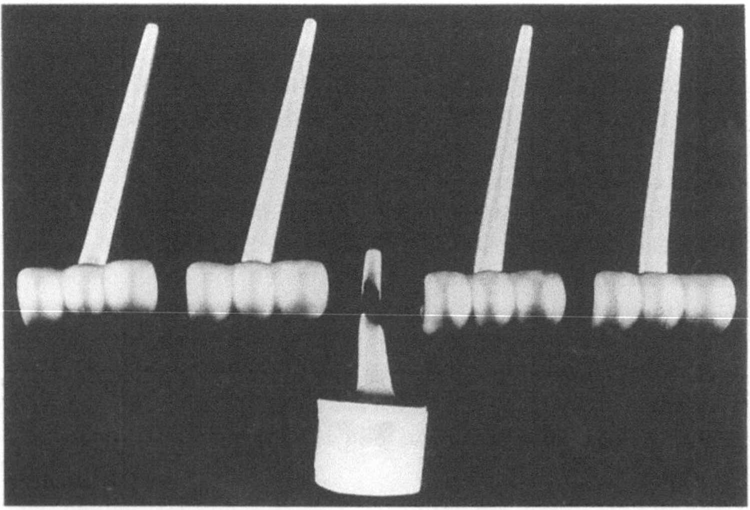

Fig. 8. The capitellocondylar implant has varying humeral angles and an anatomic restoration of the distal humerus

the ulna [12]. The bicondylar nature allows less edge loading with varus and valgus stress. The natural valgus angulation of the humerus can be restored as the distal humerus is angulated with respect to the stem. Angulation is also built into the ulnar stem. The polyethylene ulnar component is available in various thicknesses, and the stemmed humeral component is available in various angulations. These options aid in soft tissue balancing. If adequate balancing does not occur, then dislocation may result. Translocation, with the humeral component articulating at the trochleocapitellar junction, may also result due to inadequate medial tensioning (Fig. 9).

The Pritchard elbow resurfacing system (ERS) [30] prosthesis has similar mechanics, but also has the ability to be used as a cementless device (Fig. 10).

Restoration of Anatomy

Whichever implant is utilized, it is important to restore the center of rotation. This allows for better soft tissue balancing, including both the static and dynamic

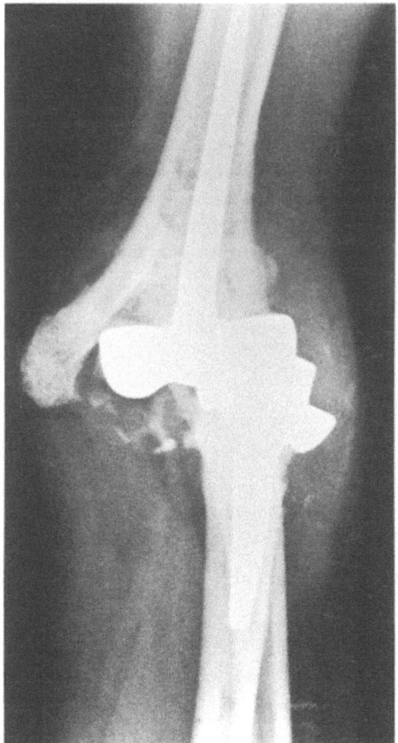

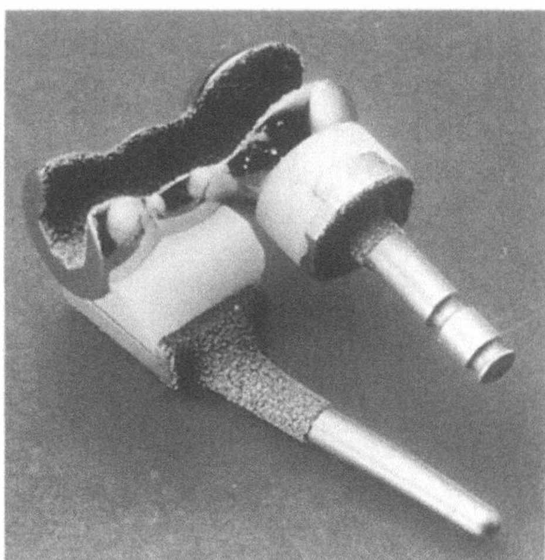

Fig. 9. If instability occurs, translocation may result, as evidenced here

Fig. 10. The Pritchard elbow resurfacing system (ERS) prosthesis has a bicondylar articulation which also allows for radial head replacement

stabilizers of the elbow. In addition, the alignment of the elbow should be restored to allow for a carrying angle so that the patient can more easily reach their face with their hand for functional activities. Restoration of anatomy may lead to a better range of motion as well as better distribution of forces. In the study of semi-constrained implants, Figgie et al. stressed the importance of restoring the center of rotation [4] (Fig. 11). The humeral center of rotation was thus placed at the natural center or in an anterior and proximal position. The acceptable position of the ulnar center of rotation was from the natural center and distal (Fig. 12). Those patients within the acceptable position had statistically better function and range of motion. In addition, there were no radiolucencies within this group. All

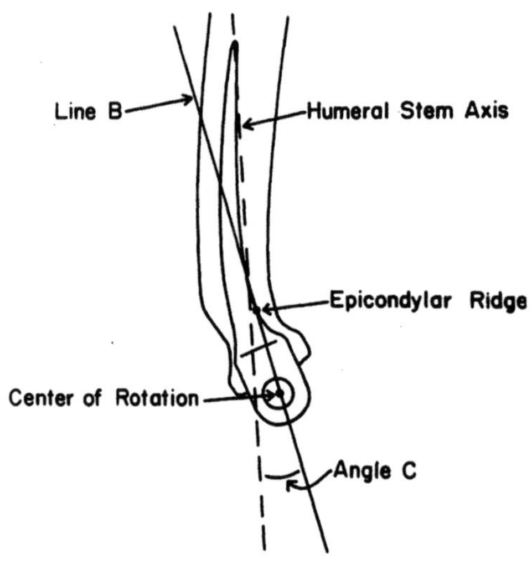

Fig. 11. The implant should restore the center of rotation (line *B*) of the natural humerus. Angle *C* represents the difference between the humeral stem axis and line B (usually 30°)

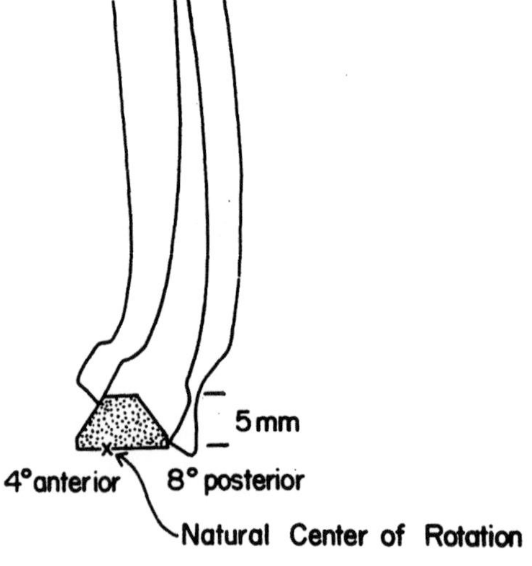

Fig. 12. The neutral zone for restoring the center of rotation is proximal to the natural center of rotation. The joint should not be elongated, as this will cause an increased joint reaction force and reduce motion

failures occurred in the elbows outside of the neutral range, including those requiring secondary procedures, dislocations, and those with lower elbow scores and less motion. Thus, any total elbow design must accurately restore the center of rotation, allow for soft tissue stabilization, and have an articulation which allows for decreased stress in the polyethylene to diminish long-term wear.

References

1. Amis AA, Dowson D, Wright V (1980) Elbow joint force predictions for some strenuous isometric actions. J Biomech 13:765–775
2. Evans EM (1945) Rotational deformity in the treatment of fractures of both bones of the forearm. J Bone Joint Surg 27:373–379
3. Ewald FC, Scheinberg RD, Poss R et al (1980) Capitellocondylar total elbow arthorplasty: two-to-five year follow-up in rheumatoid arthritis. J Bone Joint Surg 62A:1259
4. Figgie HE, Inglis AE, Moow C (1986) A critical analysis of biomechanical factors affecting functional outcome in total elbow arthorplasties. J Arthorplasty 1(3):169–173
5. Figgie MP, Inglis AE, Figgie HLE III, Mow CS (1990) Semiconstrained total elbow replacement in rheumatoid arthritis. Presentation, the 57th annual meeting of the American Academy of Orthopaedic Surgeons, New Orleans
6. Garrett JC, Ewald FC, Thomas WH, Sledge CB (1977) Loosening associated with GSB hinge total elbow replacement in patients with rheumatoid arthritis. Clin Orthop 127:170
7. Gschwend N, Loehr J, Ivosevic-Radovanovic D et al (1988) Semiconstrained elbow prostheses with special reference to the GSB III prosthesis. Clin Orthop 232:104
8. Halls AA, Travill R (1964) Transmission of pressures across the elbow-joint. Anat Rec 150:243
9. Hui FC, Chao EY, An KN (1978) Muscle and joint forces at the elbow during isometric lifting (abstract). Orthop Trans 2:169
10. Inglis AE, Pellicci PM (1980) Total elbow replacement. J Bone Joint Surg 62A:1252
11. Inglis AE (ed) (1982) Tri-axial total elbow replacement: indications, surgical technique and results. Symposium on total joint replacement of the upper extremity. Mosby, St Louis
12. Itoi E, King GJ, Morrey BF, An KN et al (1992) Stabilizers of the capitellocondylar total elbow arthroplasty. J Shoulder Elbow Surg 1:271
13. Johnson JR, Getty CJ, Mclettin AWF, Glasgow MMS (1984) The Stanmore total elbow replacement for rheumatoid arthritis. J Bone Joint Surg 66B:732
14. Kapandji IA (1970) The physiology of joints. Upper limb, 2nd edn. Williams and Wilkins, Baltimore
15. Keats TE, Teeslink R, Diamond AE, Williams JH (1966) Normal axial relationships of the major joints. Radiology 87:904–907
16. Kudo H, Iwano K, Watanabe S (1980) Total replacements of the rheumatoid elbow with a hingeless prosthesis. J Bone Joint Surg 62A:277
17. Kudo H, Iwano K (1990) Total elbow arthroplasty with a non-constrained surface replacement prosthesis in patients who have rheumatoid arthritis: a long-term follow-up study. J Bone Joint Surg 72A:355
18. London JT (1981) Kinematics of the elbow. J Bone Joint Surg 63A:529
19. Lowe LW, Miller AJ, Allum RL, Higginson DW (1984) The development of an unconstrained elbow arthroplasty: a clinical review. J Bone Joint Surg 66B:243
20. Morrey BF, Chao EYS (1976) Passive motion of the elbow joint. A biomechanical analysis. J Bone Joint Surg 58A:501–508
21. Morrey BF, Askew LJ, An KN, Chao EY (1981) A biomechanical study of normal functional elbow motion. J Bone Joint Surg 63A:872–877
22. Morrey BF, An KN (1983) Articular and ligamentous contributions to the stability of the elbow joint. Am J Sports Med 11:315

23. Morrey BF, An KN (1993) Biomechanics of the elbow. In: Morrey BF (ed) The elbow and its disorders. Saunders, Philadelphia
24. Morrey BF, An KN (1985) Functional anatomy of the elbow ligaments. Clin Orthop 201:84
25. Morrey BF, Adams RA (1992) Semiconstrained arthroplasty for the treatment of rheumatoid arthritis of the elbow. J Bone Joint Surg 74-A:479
26. O'Driscoll SW, Bell DF, Morrey BF (1991) Posterolateral rotary instability of the elbow. J Bone Joint Surg 73-A:440
27. O'Driscoll SW, An KN, Korinek S, Morrey BF (1992) Kinematics of semi-constrained total elbow arthroplasty. J Bone Joint Surg 74-B:297
28. Ogilvie WH (1930) Discussion on minor injuries of the elbow joint. Proc R Soc Med 23:306–322
29. Pearson JR, McGinley DR, Butzel LM (1963) A dynamic analysis of the upper extremity. Plantar Motions Hum. Factors 5:59
30. Pritchard RW (1983) Anatomic surface elbow arthroplasty: a preliminary report. Clin Orthop 179:223
31. Roper BA, Tuke M, O'Riordan SM, Bulstrode DJ (1986) A new unconstrained elbow. J Bone Joint Surg 68:B566
32. Schwab GH, Bennett JB, Woods GW, Tullow HS (1980) The biomechanics of elbow instability: the role of the medial collateral ligament. Clin Orthop 146:42–52
33. Soni RK, Cavendish ME (1984) A review of the Liverpool elbow prosthesis from 1974 to 1982. J Bone Joint Surg 66B:248
34. Souter WA (1981) A new approach to elbow arthroplasty. Engin Med 10(2):269
35. Spinner M, Kaplan EB (1970) The quadrate ligament of the elbow – its relationship to the stability of the proximal, radio-ulnar joint. Acta Orthop Scand 41:632–647
36. Steindler A (1977) Kinesiology of the human body, 5th edn. Thomas, Springfield
37. Tillman B (1978) A contribution to the function morphology of articular surfaces (translated by G Konorza). Thieme, Stuttgart
38. Torzilli PA (1982) Biomechanics of the elbow. In: Inglis AE (ed) Symposium on total joint replacement of the upper extremity. Mosby, St Louis
39. Wadsworth TG (1981) A new technique to total elbow replacement. Engin Med 10(2):69
40. Walker PS (1977) Human joints and their artificial replacements. Thomas, Springfield
41. Youm Y, Dryer RF, Thambyrajah K et al (1979) Biomechanical analysis of forearm pronation-supination and elbow flexion-extension. J Biomech 12:245–255

Non-Endoprosthetic Procedures

Arthroscopy of the Elbow

C. Jantea, W. Rüther, and A. Baltzer

Introduction

Arthroscopy of the elbow is a promising technique for enlarging the surgical spectrum in treating various pathological conditions of the elbow [1, 2]. Arthroscopy of the elbow should be performed only after having obtained all relevant information by noninvasive diagnostic evaluation. Therefore arthroscopy is considered to be a surgical technique exclusively [3]. When performing arthroscopy, The surgical anatomy of the elbow must be respected meticulously to avoid iatrogenic lesions [4]. This chapter describes the surgical technique for arthroscopic treatment of elbow pathology.

Preoperative Diagnosis, Indication for Arthroscopy, and Patient Selection

The patient's history and a very careful clinicial examination are the prerequisites for establishing the diagnosis [5]. Several diagnostic procedures are available, but noninvasive ones should be preferred [3]. For detecting bony pathology one should start with the X-ray examination in standard views: AP view with the elbow extended, lateral view with the elbow flexed at 90° in neutral rotation, and AP view with the elbow in 45° of internal and external rotation. The X-ray examination should be followed by computed tomography and magnetic resonance imaging in cases in which the diagnosis is still doubtful after the X-ray examination alone. Bone scan performed in the three-phase technique offers the advantage of differentiating between bony and soft tissue pathology. Magnetic resonance imaging is very helpful in diagnosing soft tissue changes around the elbow. Floursocopy and kinematography may be helpful in the documenting the instability pattern of the elbow. Sonography, thermography, and arthrography are not useful techniques for the diagnosis of elbow pathology.

The aim of the extensive preoperative examination of the elbow is to distinguish between intra- and extra-articular pathology. Only intra-articular conditions of the elbow can be treated by the arthroscopic technique. Selected extra-articular pathologic changes may be treated endoscopically, for example, decompression of the ulnar nerve at the cubital tunnel [6] and the release of extensor aponeurosis in the so-called "tennis elbow" [7]. Intra-articular conditions can be divided into changes concerning the soft tissue (synovitis, intra-articular bands, posttraumatic contracture of the capsule) and those of the bony structures (chondromatosis, loose bodies, flake fractures, fracture with an osteochondral fragment, osteochondrosis dissecans, osteoarthrosis with degeneration of the cartilage, formation of osteophytes). It is important to realize before arthroscopy that the proximal radioulnar joint can be visualized only in part both from the anterior and from the posterior [4].

The general contraindications for general anesthesia should be respected in patients with cardiac and pulmonary disease. Arthroscopy of the elbow is performed in brachial plexus anesthesia or in an intravenous regional block (Bier's block). Absolute contraindications are lesion of the skin and previous operations with reconstruction or transposition of the nerves, for example, the ulnar nerve. Relative contraindications include severe joint contractures that do not allow distenting the joint capsule and bony ancylosis.

Surgical Technique

Surgical procedures can be divided into reconstructive and symptomatic techniques. Reconstructive techniques aim to restore the anatomic intact joint, for example, arthroscopically assisted reduction of intra-articular fractures. Palliative or symptomatic techniques aim to eliminate the factors inducing the dysfunction of the joint, for example, abrasion arthroplasty in osteoarthritis and synovectomy in rheumatoid arthritis.

Arthroscopy of the elbow is usually performed with the patient in supine position (Fig. 1). In this position there is no technical limitation for the arthroscopic portals. Furthermore, if arthrotomy of the joint is required, this can easily be performed while the arm is positioned on an armtable after removing the arthroscopic equipment. Another atvantage of the supine position is the fact that motion in the shoulder joint is not restricted, thus allowing any position of the arm as required during surgery. To avoid iatrogenic lesions of the intra-articular structures we recommend performing arthroscopy of the elbow in a sitting set-up for the surgeons and the assisting nurse. The assistant and the surgeon should have the same view on the monitor. Surgery can also be observed by the patient on the same monitor as the surgeon, as arthroscopy of the elbow can be performed in plexus anaesthesia with the patient in supine position (Fig. 1). The arthroscopic instruments should be adapted for the elbow. Usually the diameter of the instruments should not be greater than 3.5 mm.

Arthroscopic Portals to the Elbow

Two portals are necessary to perform a surgical intervention arthroscopically at the elbow. The arthroscope is introduced through one portal; the second portal

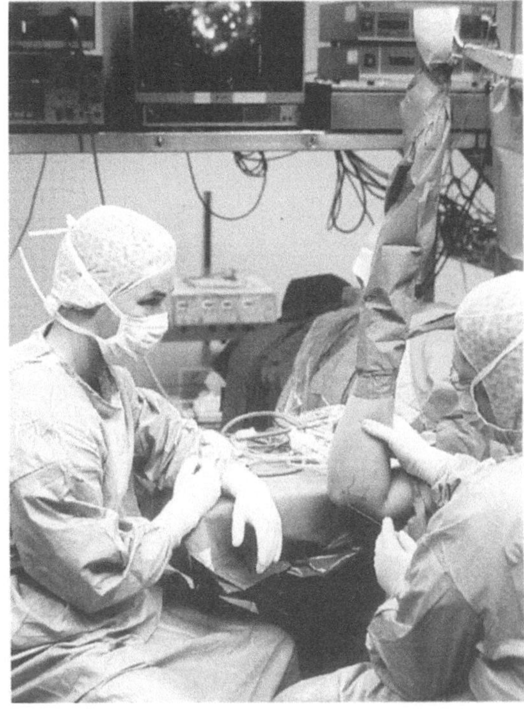

Fig. 1. Arthroscopy of the elbow is performed with the patient in supine position and under plexus anesthesia. The arm is fixed by a device which does not limit the motion of the joint. The patient, surgeon, and nurse can observe surgery on the same monitor. The arthroscopic instruments are placed on a separate table (not on the patient)

may be used to introduce instruments into the joint and to perform intra-articular manipulation under direct visualization (Fig. 2a,b). The arthroscopic portals pass through muscles and close to nerve structures, and the preoperative diagnosis must therefore be precise as one may use only the portal necessary to treat the intra-articular pathology [2, 4]. Lesions of the cutaneous nerves can be avoided if the subcutaneous tissue is spread carefully with a blunt clamp after the skin incision.

The radial head and humeroradial joint line are the bony landmarks for placement of the lateral portals. First, the joint is inflated by the posterolateral portal, with the elbow flexed at 90° in neutral rotation of the forearm. Then a spinal needle is introduced into the anterolateral portal, and the outflow of the intra-articular fluid is observed if the anterolateral portal is in the correct position (Figs. 2a,b, 3). The anterior joint compartment is usually visualized through the anterolateral portal (Figs. 2b, 4). For surgery one may establish a second anterolateral portal, which should be located in 3–4 cm distance from the first one. The anteromedial portal is used if the arthroscope must be switched from medial to lateral when performing intra-articular manipulations (Figs. 2a,b, 5). In this situation one may use the so-called Wissinger rod when changing the instruments (Fig. 2c,d).

The anterior part of the joint can be visualized using the anterolateral and anteromedial portals, and the proximal radioulnar joint can be seen in part

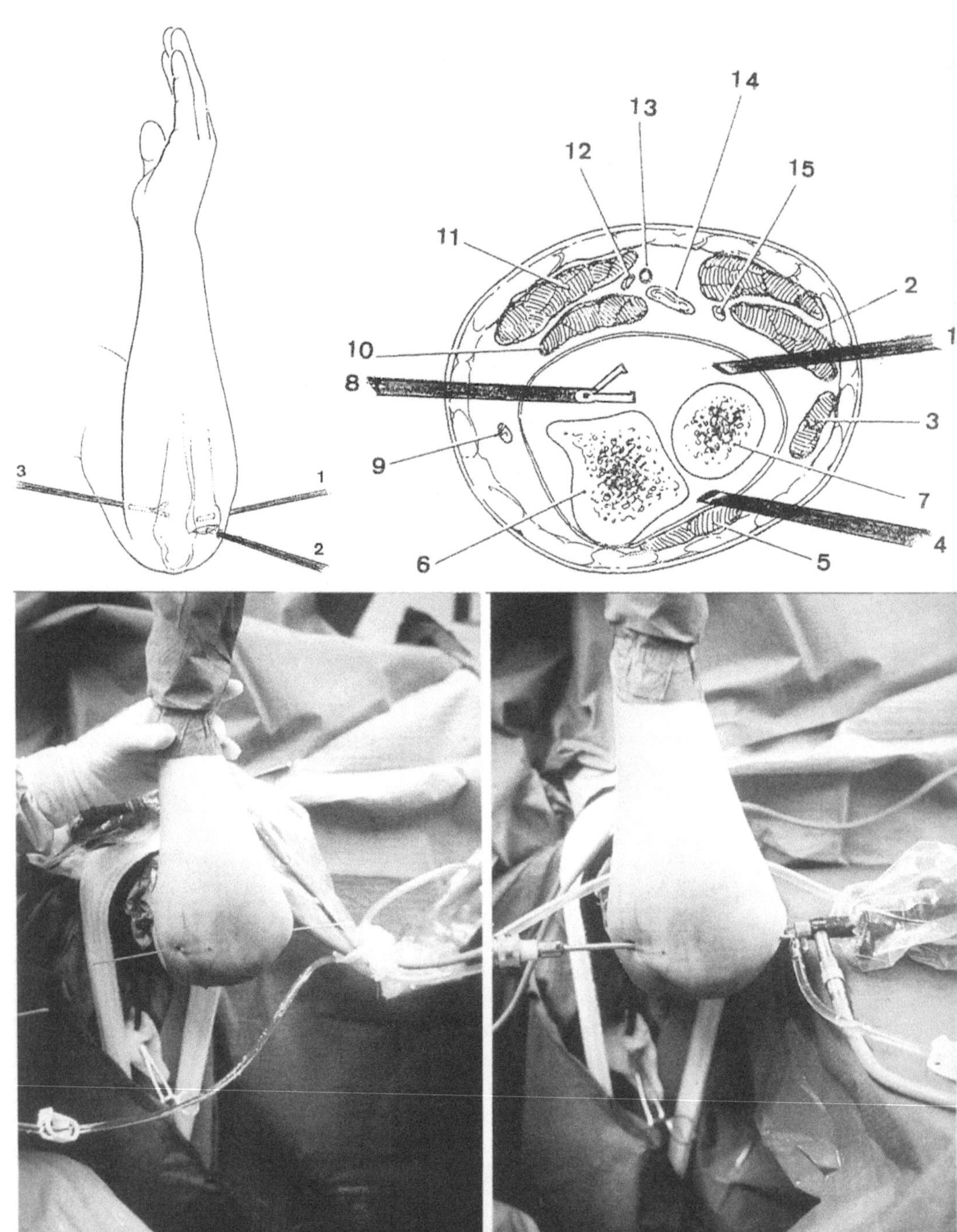
13
14
12
15
11
2
10
1
8
3
9
7
6
4
5
a
c
3
1
2

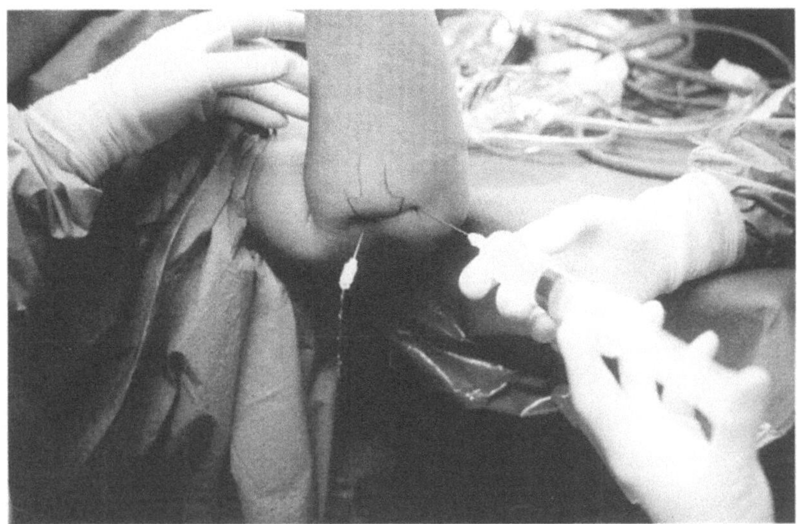

Fig. 3. The joint is inflated through the posterolateral portal in neutral position of the joint. With a spinal needle in the anterolateral portal the best position for this apporach is tested before the skin incision is made

through the anterior and the posterolateral portal (Fig. 6). The posterolateral portal is established lateral to the aponeurosis of the triceps muscle for visualization. The working cannula is introduced into the joint through the posterocentral or a second posterolateral portal. Accessory portals should be avoided to diminish the risk of neurovascular lesions. A miniarthrotomy, for example, when removing free bodies, may be necessary; therefore the arthroscopic portal should be positioned in line with potential open surgical approaches to the joint.

Fig. 2. a View of the elbow joint with the standard portals: *1*, anterolateral; *2*, posterolateral; *3*, anteromedial. (Modified after [9]) **b** Transverse section of the elbow show the relative position of the portals in the joint. The anterolateral portal penetrates the extensor digit. com. (*2*) and extensor carpi rad. (*3*) muscles. The posterolateral portal (*4*) passes throught the acnoneuas muscle (*5*). Through this portal the dorsal aspect of the radial head (*7*) and the olecranon (*6*) can be visualized. The anteromedial portal (*8*) passes before the ulnar nerve (*9*). Continuous intra-articular irrigation is necessary to inhibit collapse of the anterior joint capsule and to avoid lesions of the brachial (*10*) and pronator teres (*11*) muscles, median nerve (*12*), brachial arterey (*13*), tendon of the biceps muscle (*14*), and the radial nerve (*15*). (Modified after [9]) **c** View of a right elbow with the switching stick (Wissinger rod) positioned intra-articulary in the anterior joint compartment. Over the rod the cannulas for the instruments can be changed from medial to lateral and changing the position of the arthroscope from the anterolateral in the anteromedial portal. **d** View on the motorized shaver in the anterolateral portal. The arm can be stabilized with a weight of 2 kg without limitation of the joint motion

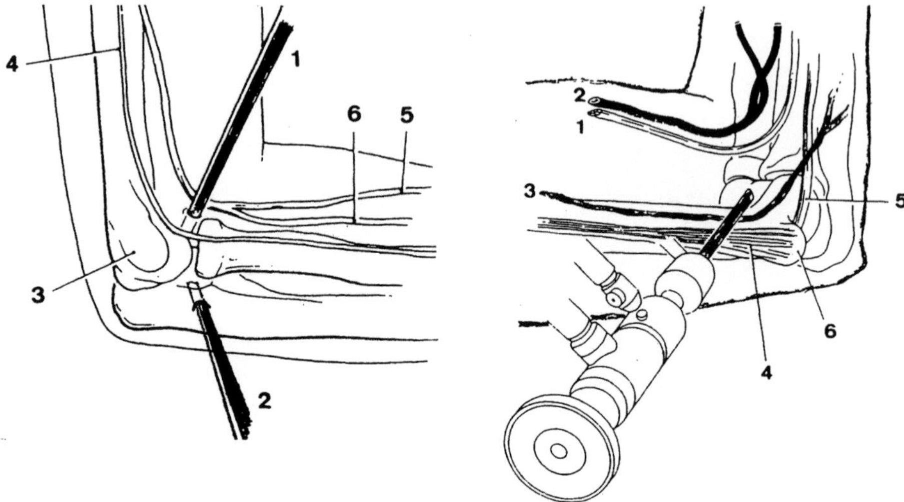

Fig. 4. Scheme of the anterolateral (*1*) and posterolateral (*2*) portal. These portals are introduced after exact identification of the radial head and the lateral epicondyle (*3*) by palpation. The portals are located anterior and posterior to the lateral collateral ligament. The anterior joint compartment and a segment of the proximal radioulnar joint can be visualized through these portals. Lesions of the n. cutaneus antebrachii lateralis (*4*), radial nerve with its superficial (*5*), and deep motor branch (*6*) should be avoided by gentle placements of the portals. (Modified after [9])

Fig. 5. Scheme of the anteromedial portal. The anterior part of the humeroulnar joint can be visualized through this portal. The portal is established in the inside-out technique after positioning of the anterolateral portal. By distension of the joint capsule lesions of the median nerve (*1*) and the brachial artery (*2*) can be avoided. The medial antebrachial cutaneus nerve (*3*) is located anterior to the intermuscular septum (*4*). The ulnar nerve (*5*) lies in its canal protected by the medial epicondyle (*6*). (Modified after [9])

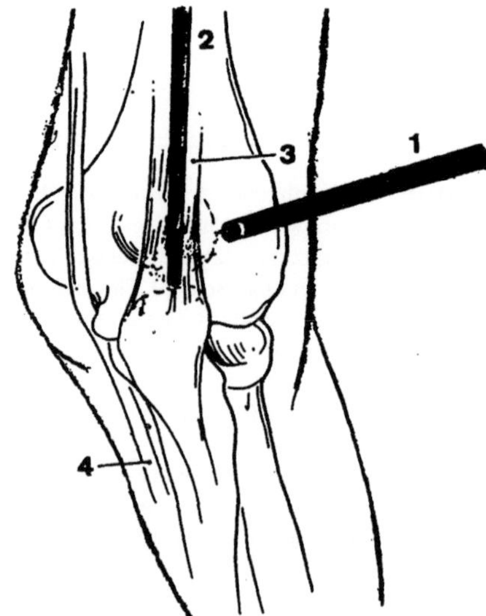

Fig. 6. View of the elbow with the standrard portals in the posterior joint compartment. The posterolateral portal (*1*) is positioned ca. 3 cm proximal to the leteral epicondyle. The posterocentral portal (*2*) passes the triceps muscle (*3*). Portals in the medial aspect of the dorsal joint compartment should be avoided as the ulnar nerve (*4*) could be at risk. (Modified after [9])

Technical Mistakes, Complications, and Results

On the basis of precise preoperative planning a decision is made before surgery as to what portals are necessary to treat the specific joint pathology. One should avoid establishing all standard portals in a routine way. One of the disadvantages is that a joint compression can occur by the extravasation of fluid, and that the arthroscopic procedure must be finished before surgery [2]. A cannula should always be left in place after establishing the portal; tissue traumatization can thus be avoided as the portals pass through muscle. The Wissinger rod must fit precisely in the cannula, thus avoiding squeezing of the soft tissue between the cannula and the rod (Fig. 2c,d). The routine use of a pump to maintain constant pressure should be avoided as great volumes can flow outside the joint between the capsule and the skin and result in an extra-articular joint compression, which might compromise the view inside the joint. If a pump is used, one should start with a low pressure of 40–60 mmHG.

Arthroscopy of the elbow is a very demanding technique, and many details must be strictly respected. When several surgeons are performing the arthroscopy, the incidence of complications can be as high as 20% [8]. If, hovever, the arthroscopic education is standardized, for example, quality control after surgery in anatomic specimens and artificial joint models, assistance of experienced surgeons, the iatrogenic complication rate can be reduced significantly. At the Orthopedic Department of the Heinrich Heine University no complications due to the surgical technique have been observed after introducion of a strict curriculum for surgeons performing elbow surgery and arthroscopy.

Several complications have been described for general arthroscopy which may also occur at the elbow. However, one must distinguish between specific and general complications. Specific complications are related to the arthroscopic technique, for example, lesions of cartilage and bone when establishing the portals and lesions of the periarticular nerves by penetration of the joint capsule [9, 15, 16]. Nerve lesions must be avoided because neural regeneration is limited around the elbow due to the great relative motion and gliding distances of the nerves during flexion and extension motion of the elbow, and because more extensive secondary procedures are required to restore the function of the arm and hand after lesions to the main nerves of the arm [10–14]. General complications as in other surgical procedures (e.g., infection, excessive scaring) can also occur in elbow arthroscopy [1, 16]. Thrombosis of the arm veins and necrosis of the soft tissue around the portals with joint fistulas can be observed if the protal is too large and is not sutured after surgery [2].

The following pathologic conditions can be treated sucessfully and are good indications for arthroscopy. The first is removal of free or loose bodies (Fig. 7); in most cases these are located in the dorsal humeroradial joint where they can be easily found and removed [18]. Arthroscopy is established as a standard procedure in patients with rheumatoid arthritis due to the polyarticular course of the disease; therefore minimally invasive surgery, performed effectively, may be helpful in avoiding multiple scars. However, as in other joints, we have shown in an experimental study that complete synovectomy of the joint is technically not possible through the standard arthroscopic portals. Around 15% residual synovia were found after both arthroscopic synovectomy and synovectomy through the bilateral approach [17]. Under clinical circumstances one must therefore consider the possibility of performing a radiosynoviorthesis after the arthroscopic procedure, thus avoiding recurrence of the disease from residual synovia. Follow-up of arthroscopic joint débridement shows good results in ostearthotic joints [2]. In posttraumatic changes arthroscopy should be performed as the first procedure before further surgery is indicated (Fig. 7a).

Arthroscopy can be used to assist the reduction of intra-articular fractures and to wash out intra-articular hematoma. The technique is very demanding as it

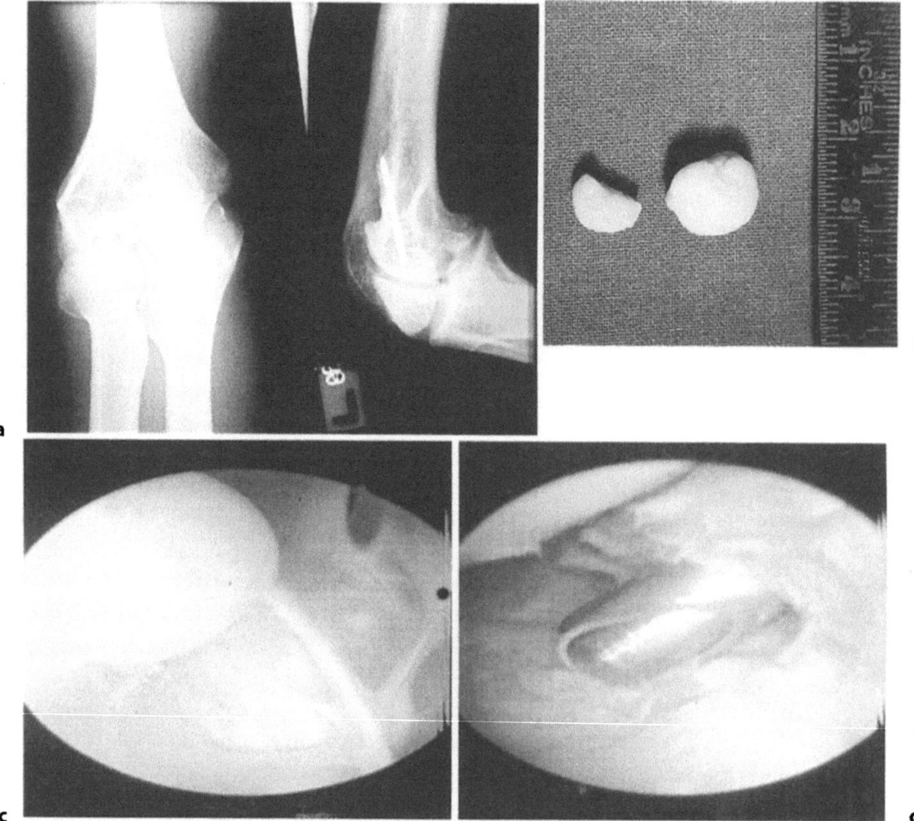

Fig. 7. a Posttraumatic arthrosis in a 30-year-old patient after fracture of the distal humerus with loose bodies, which could not be visualized radiologically. **b** Loose bodies after removal. The arthroscopic portal had to be slightly enlarged to extract the loose bodies out of the joint. **c** Arthroscopic view of the loose body in the anterior joint compartment. **d** Synovitis accompanying slight chondral degeneration of the cartilage of the humeroradial joint segment is débrided using a synovial resector

requires in addition to the arthroscopic equipment an X-ray image intensifier to control the result of reposition and fragment fixation. Arthroscopy can be recommended in simple fractures without comminution, for example, of the radial head. In acute situations one must consider that a lesion of the joint capsule has probably also occurred; therefore arthroscopic surgery must be very early to avoid extravasation of the fluid. In patients with osteochondrosis dissecans arthroscopic treatment may be indicated by preoperative investigation performed by magnetic resonance imaging. If the cartilage is intact, retrograde drilling is recommended to penetrate the avascular zone. Fixation with biodegrable pins is recommended if sparation of the osteochondral fragment is probable. In the case of a loose body open surgery is performed because the technical limitation of the arthroscopic instruments at this time makes the arthroscopical refixation of loose fragments at the elbow too time consuming (Fig. 8).

Defining the role of arthroscopy at the elbow is very difficult. Publications report the authors' experiences with this technique and describe technical

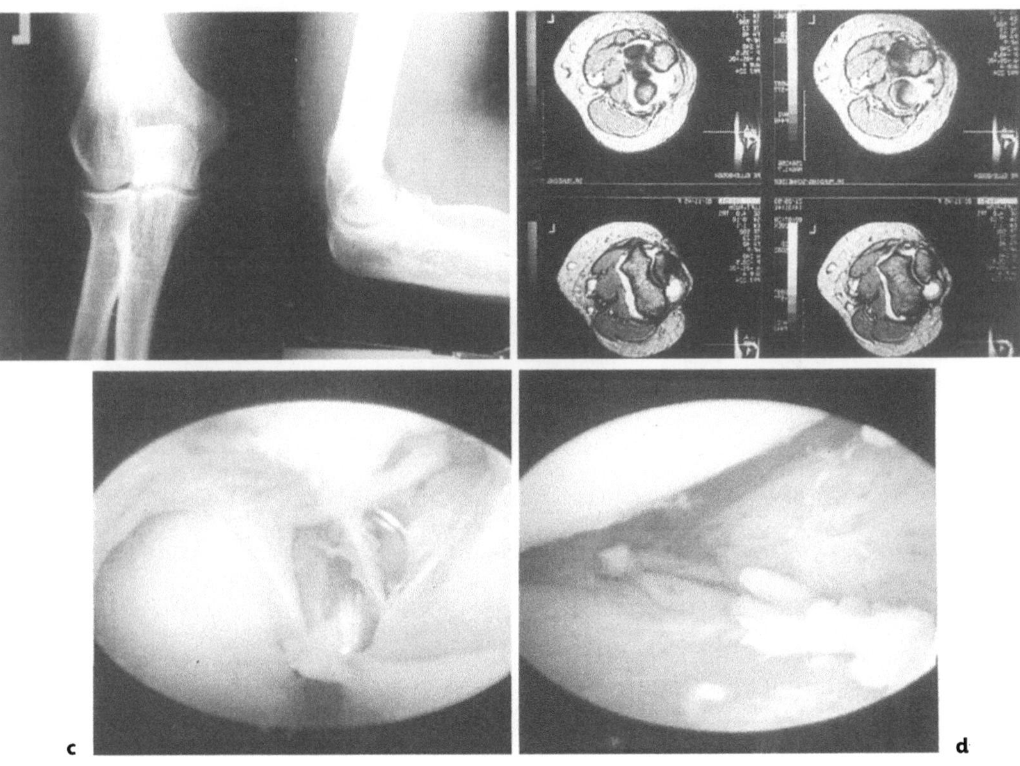

Fig. 8. a Seronegative monarthritis in a 45-year-old patient. Clinically there is concentric limitation of movement, but no changes are seen in the joint at radiological examination (stage 0-I according to Larsen). b Magnetic resonance imaging shows an intra-articular effusion and synovitis localized preferentially in the humeroradial joint segment. c Arthroscopic view of the radiohumeral joint segment with synovitis and intra-articular development of adhesions. d Arthroscopic view of the posterolateral segment of the radiohumeral joint with localized synovitis

details. There are no studies comparing patients treated arthroscopically to those treated by the standard technique in open surgery. Furthermore, as all possible diagnoses are reported, one cannot distinguish in the follow-up reports the role of the arthroscopic procedure in a specific diagnosis by a strict classification concerning the stage of the disease. However, most authors confirm the advantages of arthroscopy demonstrated at other joint locations, for example, minimal surgical portals, shorter postoperative rehabilitation, less pain postoperatively, reduction in invalides, and lower costs. However, only a prospective study comparing the same patient population after treatment by arthroscopicy and by open surgery can confirm these presumed advantages of arthroscopy.

Summary

Arthroscopy of the elbow should be perfomed only as a surgical technique, as other imaging techniques are available to establish the diagnosis. Iatrogeneic complications can be avoided by strictly respecting the technical recommendations and the topographic anatomy of the joint. In selected indications, such as removal of loose bodies, arthroscopy has a defined role as a minimally invasive surgical technique.

References

1. Andrews JR, Pierre S, Carson W (1986) Arthroscopy of the elbow. Clin Sports Med 5:653–662
2. O'Driscoll SW, Morrey BF (1994) Arthroscopy of the elbow. In: Morrey BF (ed) The elbow – master techniques in orthopedic surgery. Raven, New York, pp 27–34
3. Jantea C, Rüther W, Assheuer J (1995) Stellenwert der bildgebenden Verfahren am Ellenbogengelenk. Arthroskopie (in press)
4. Jantea C (1992) Arthroscopy of the elbow. Karl Storz Company Videotheque, Tuttlingen, Germany
5. Lewit K (1992) Manuelle Medizin. Urban & Schwarzenberg, Munich
6. Tsai TM (1994) Endoscopic therapy of the cubital tunnel syndrom. In: Proceedings of the Federation of the European Societies for Surgery of the Hand Conference, Dublin, June
7. Krämer J (1993) Endoskopische Therapie der Epikondylopathie des Ellenbogens 6:272–273
8. Jerosch J, Drescher H, Steinbeck J, Schröder M (1994) Arthroskopie des Ellenbogengelenks. Indikationen, Ursachen von neurologischen Komplikationen, Prävention. Arthroskopie 7:25–33
9. McGinty JB (ed) (1991) Operative arthroscopy, Raven, New York
10. Lundborg G (1988) Nerve injury and repair. Churchill Livingstone, New York
11. Millesi H (1992) Chirurgie der peripheren Nerven. Urban & Schwarzenberg, Munich
12. Gelberman RH (ed) (1991) Opertive nerve repair and reconstruction. Lippincott, Philadelphia
13. Mackinnon SE, Dellon AL (1988) Surgery of the peripheral nerve. Thieme, Stuttgart
14. Sunderland S (1991) Nerve injuries and their repair. Churchill Livingstone, New York
15. Papilion J, Neff R, Shall L (1988) Compression neuropathy of the radial nerve as a complication of elbow arthroscopy: a case report and review of the literature. Arthroscopy 4:284–286
16. O'Driscoll SW, Morrey BF (1992) Arthroscopy of the elbow: diagnostic and therapeutic benefits and hazards. J Bone Joint Surg Am 74:84–94

17. Jantea C, Jerosch J, Castro W (1989) Synovectomy of the elbow – open surgery versus arthroscopic procedure (an experimental study). Proceedings of the European Rheumatoid Arthritis Surgical Societies, Congress. Bürgenstock, Switzerland
18. Guhl JF (1985) Arthroscopy and arthroscopic surgery of the elbow. Orthopedics 8:1290–1296

Late Synovectomy of the Elbow Joint

A. Wanivenhaus and W. Bretschneider

Introduction

In 21%–68% of cases, the elbow joint is involved in rheumatoid arthritis (RA) [1–4]. Only in rare cases, i.e., 1.7%–3% [5, 6], does the disease start at this joint. At the time of initiation of treatment, the initial stage of rheumatoid arthritis is long over [7] and, according to Gschwend [2], distinct signs of destruction can be observed in 70% of the patients. As the elbow is located in the middle of a series of joints, it is of considerable importance. Therefore, many procedures have been developed for its surgical treatment.

Therapy by synoviorthesis was followed by synovectomy with or without resection of the radial head, resection arthroplasty, and endoprostheses, which are now well-established, partially complementary, and partially parallel methods [8].

In the present paper we restrict the indication for synovectomy to cases with an advanced degree of destruction (Larsen stage 3 and above) [9] and compare it with reports in the literature. Early synovectomy undoubtedly gives better results and has to be regarded as an optimal form of therapy. It is reported that more than 70% of patients are satisfied with the outcome of this surgery or could be ameliorated, whereas late synovectomy shows a success rate of less than 70% [10, 11], which could be shown to decrease with increasing follow-up to values as low as 37% after 12 years, as reported by Vahvanen et al. [11] They advocate the opinion that the increasing dissatisfaction with the outcome of the surgery is due to bone loss and resulting instability. Tressel thinks the dissatisfaction might be due to increasing secondary arthrosis [12]. Some authors are of opinion that resection of the radial head might also be responsible for the occurrence of instabilities [13–16], whereas others could not find any difference when they directly compared patients with and without resection of the radial head [17, 18]. Grimm did not even notice an increase in instability after more than 5 years of follow-up [19]. Similarly, Eichenblat did not find a significant difference between patients with long and short follow-up periods [20]. Copeland [17] does not distinguish between low-grade and high-grade destruction of the joint and does not find differences in instability of joints with or without resection of the radial head, therefore pleading for maintenance of the radial head. However, the same author reports to have performed subsequent resection of the radial head in two patients to ensure adequate rotation and flexion. However, Taylor distinctly recommends resection of the radial head and did not observe a considerable increase in instability [21]. Eichenblat [20] points out that 20 of 25 patients underwent simultaneous resection of the distal ulna within the wrist, thereby avoiding length discrepancies between radius and ulna. In his study Porter [4] shows the discrepancies in evaluation of the patients' satisfaction depending on the parameter included in the calculation (subjective satisfaction alone or combined with surgical evaluation and with or without radiological evaluation). Consideration of the mentioned parameters leads to a decrease in satisfaction from 71% to 63% and even 54.4%.

According to Morrey [22], a functional range of motion of 90° flexion and 100° rotation (50° each for pronation and supination) is the minimum clinical result required for the surgical method to be judged successful. The data on 1085 elbow joints (1011 synovectomies) given in 19 references published between 1971 and 1991 [4, 7, 8, 10–12, 15, 17–21, 24, 30–36] (551 of which can be defined as late synovectomies) show an average range of motion of the elbow joint of 119° flexion (22.5° extension deficit) and 140° of rotation (pronation/supination). Simultaneously, an amelioration of the subjective condition is stated after a mean of 5.1 years of follow-up in 79% of the cases (range, 67% [10]–100% [20]), which clearly indicates that the surgical method gives good functional results and the outcome leads to subjective satisfaction of the patients.

The initial situation of this group of patients seems clear and homogenous: increasing pain even without load at minimum motion mainly within the humeroradial part of the joint, extension deficit, but in most cases still a flexion of more than 100°. Limitation of rotation is observed only after the appearance of an extension deficit and is finally accompanied by an increasing inhibition of flexion [2]. The residual flexibility and the present stability may be the reasons for the late observance of a functional deficit which leads to surgical intervention, a possible explanation for the considerable number of late synovectomies.

Material and Method

Between 1985 and 1991 in our department 19 patients suffering from rheumatoid arthritis (22 elbow joints) with advanced degree of destruction (Larsen stages 3 and 4) were treated. A total of 15 patients with an average follow-up of 4.2 years could be investigated clinically, and in three cases the data could be collected from the patients' history. One patient had already died; however, X-rays and function of the elbow joint of this patient had been documented, enabling us to report on all patients.

Mean age at surgery was 51 years (range, 21–78 years); 18 patients were women and four were men. Surprisingly, the dominant arm was not affected in the majority of cases: all patients were right-handers, but only in nine cases was the right elbow joint concerned.

All patients but one suffered from pain (however, 35% of the patients only low-grade pain), synovitis, and distinct pressure pain over the humeroradial joint.

Only 40% of the patients were able to perform everyday movements such as combing their hair, eating, dressing, washing, and throwing of an object with the affected arm. Symptoms of the ulnar nerve were observed only in two patients in whom a ventral dislocation was performed from an additional ulnar approach.

The initial radiologic situation was Larsen stage 3 in all but five patients; these five presented with Larsen stage 4.

The preoperative range of flexion was 104° and the extension deficit was 24°. Range of rotation was 127° (61.7° pronation and 66° supination). Especially active and passive rotation in the sense of supination was highly painful in the terminal position.

We chose a radial surgical approach in all patients except for two who underwent additional dislocation of the ulnar nerve. The radial head was resected in all but one patient under special consideration of maintenance of the stability of the radioulnar ligament. All osteophytes inhibiting flexion or extension were resected until only healthy material appeared. Thereafter, the bone spongiosa wounds were closed with bone wax. Resection of lateral osteophytes was performed with caution. In the case of extension deficits, we performed additional ventral loosening of the capsule; in the case of a tendency towards a valgus position, additional loosening of the extensors was necessary. Our aim was a maximally movable elbow joint primarily free of tensions. The joint is fixed via a dorsal plaster cast for the upper arm at a neutral position of the lower arm until removal of the drains. According to the pain status of the patient, active or passive mobilization of the flexion is started, which can be followed by passive rotation after good tolerance of the initial exercises.

Results

With a rate of amelioration of 91%, the subjective satisfaction with this method can be judged as excellent. The same percentage of patients would agree to undergo this method of surgery again. Subjective satisfaction with the function of the joint was significantly better, and in all cases but one patients were able to perform all movements necessary for everyday life with the operated joint.

Moreover, a significant reduction in pain was achieved with this surgery: 14 patients were pain free and only two patients complained of considerable pain, which, however, was less pronounced than prior to surgery.

The range of motion was 110°. Total flexion increased from 104° preoperatively to 125° postoperatively (range, 100°–140°). The extension deficit decreased from 24° preoperatively to 18.5° postoperatively (range, 0°–35°). The mean rotation after surgery was 154.2° as compared to 127° prior to surgery, with a supination of 75.7° almost equal to pronation (78.5°). In our patients no case of serious instability was observed (Table 1).

As expected, radiologic evaluation showed worsening of the stage. Whereas preoperatively 17 patients showed stage III and five patients stage IV, we observed

Table 1. Range of movement ($n = 22$)

	Preoperative	Postoperative
Flexion	104°	125°
Extension deficit	24°	18.5°
Rotation		
Pronation	61.7°	78.5°
Supination	66°	75.7°

Table 2. Isometric measurement (mean values) using a Loredan work-set

	Operation group	Control group
Extension (Nm)	14.4	19.8
Flexion (Nm)	17.5	21.2
Pronation (Ncm)	262.2	248.5
Supination (Ncm)	288.5	252

stage III in 12 cases, stage IV in eight cases, and stage V in two cases after surgery (Fig. 1). The two elbow joints judged stage V were those of a female patient with juvenile rheumatoid arthritis who had been operated on both arms. The diagnosis of all other patients was rheumatoid arthritis.

We performed measurement of isometric force using a Loredan (West Sacramento, CA, USA) work-set, resulting in 17.5 Nm (flexion) and 14.4 Nm (extension), respectively. This shows a postoperatively decreased force in flexion movement due to resection of the radial head (the respective values for comparable nonoperated patients are: flexion, 21.2 Nm; extension, 19.8 Nm). However, this is compensated by a significantly increased force and range of rotation movement (pronation 262.2 Ncm and supination 288.5 Ncm in the operated group as compared to 248.5 Ncm and 252 Ncm, respectively, in nonoperated patients). These findings are in good correlation with those reported by Vahvanen [11] (Table 2).

Discussion

As stated by Torgerson [31], synovectomy sooner or later results in a significant decrease in pain and an acceptable range of motion. This is confirmed by our investigations. Surgery brought about a considerable gain in function by increased mobility. Subjective satisfaction and acceptance were stated by 90% of the patients and surmounted our expectations by far. However, it must be pointed out that radiologic investigations showed worsening which after a long follow-up may lead to bone resorption and instability caused by secondary arthrosis [12] or by resection of the radial head.

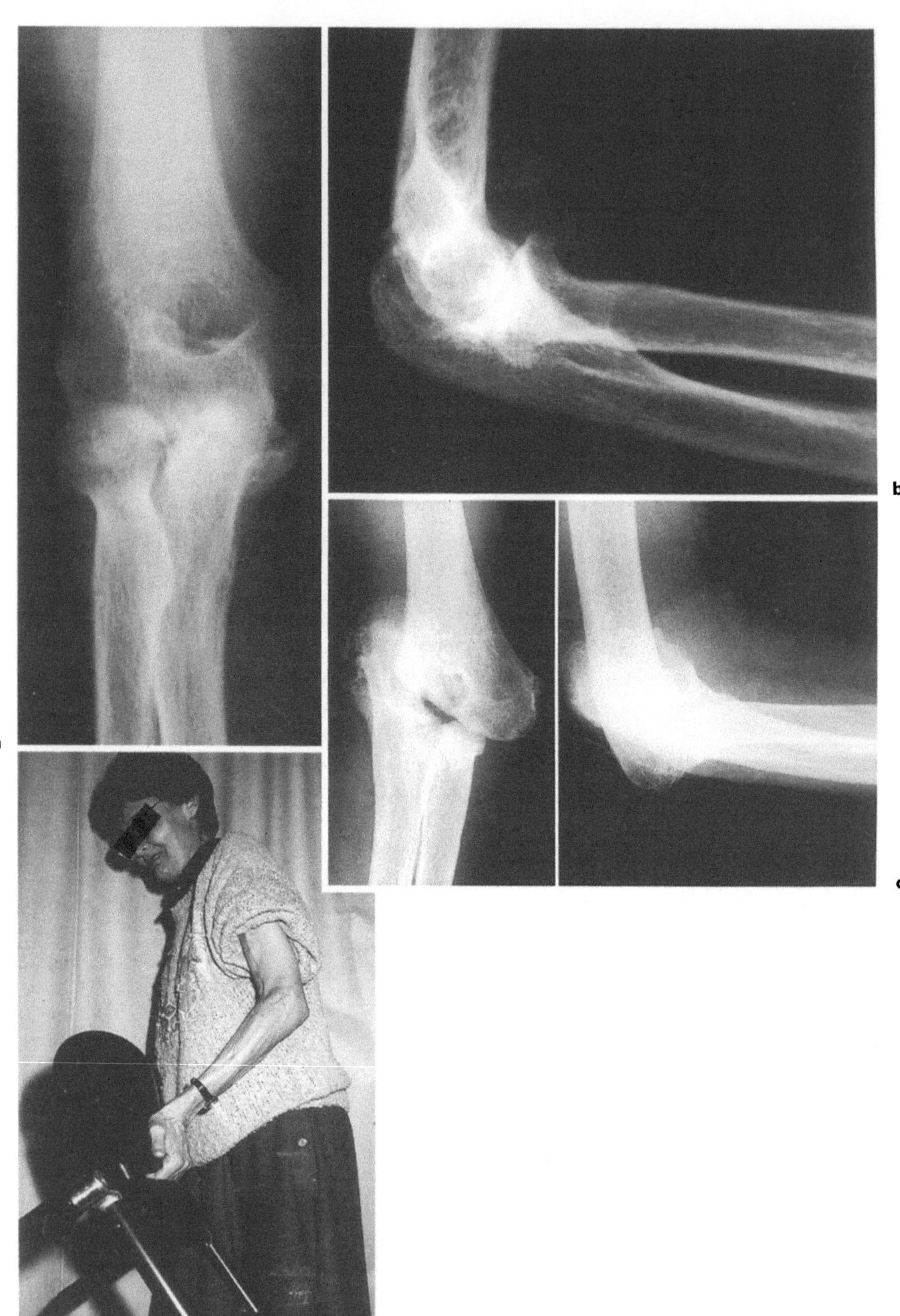

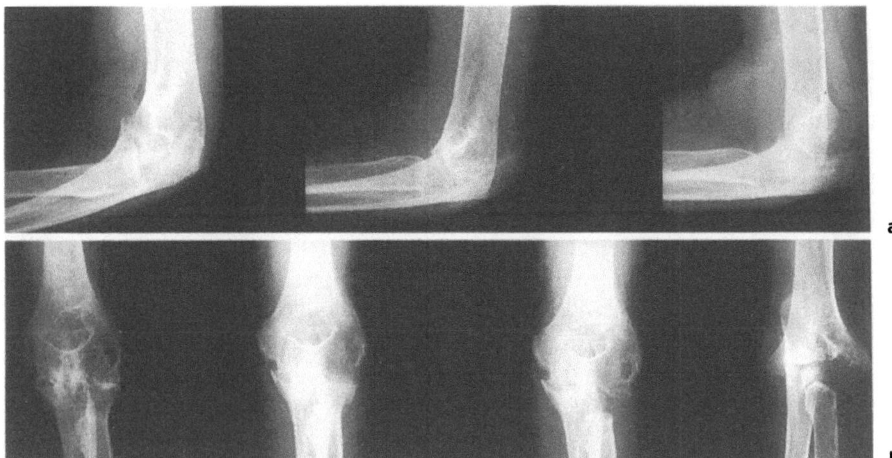

Fig. 2a,b. Female patient born in 1922. Course during 8 years. Despite resection of the radial head, no valgus position of the elbow joint

In our patients we did not observe an appreciable increase in instability (in the sense of valgus position) after resection of the radial head (Fig. 2). In two cases we had the impression of a varus position caused by narrowing of the humeroulnar part of the joint. However, no definite conclusion can be drawn from this limited number of patients as to whether the extended debridement with removal of the capsule and extensor was successful or whether follow-up is still too short. Saito [24], too, extended surgery to extensive debridement of the joint and complete removal of the extensor or even to complete capsulotomy and also reported amelioration in 90% of the cases after a mean follow-up of 4 years. Siekmann [19] did not observe increased instability in a long-term study, but significantly better values for pronation and supination. Resection of the radial head proves useful after long-term follow-up merely by an increased range of rotation. Tressel [12] states the problem of an increased instability due to resection of the radial head; however, he had to resect the radial head in all cases during a second operation and therefore recommends primary resection.

Vahvanen [11] observed decreasing satisfaction and considerable bone destruction, though without a loss in the range of motion. Therefore, a good functional result was observed even after long-term follow-up. After a follow-up of more than 10 years, Tressel [12] is of opinion that function can be ameliorated during the late stage from a long-term point of view. Tulp [8] did not observe a significant difference between early and late synovectomy in his patients after a follow-up of 6.5 and 8.5 years, respectively, and he therefore prefers the method

Fig. 1a–d. Female patient born in 1932. Significant worsening of an initial Larsen stage 4. Flexion 35°-10°-0°, pronation 40°-0°-30°. Subjective satisfaction with the result 5 years postoperatively over implantation of a prosthesis, even in cases with extensive osseous destructions.

In the majority of patients the radial approach is sufficient. In none of our patients with extensive destruction of the joint were we able to save the radial head, and therefore an extended approach as proposed by Böhler [31] and Gschwend [32] was not necessary. Only in a case of marked irritation of the ulnar nerve was its reposition performed via a second ulnar approach [33, 34].

Performance of interposition arthroplasty of the radial head using Silastic (Dow Corning, Midland, MI, USA) [35], as recommended by several authors as a short-term solution, has to be refused nowadays.

It should be pointed out that especially in an advanced stage we performed resection of the distal ulna in the course of synovectomy of the hand joint – a primary Darrach procedure even recommended by Marmor [7], who achieved excellent results in his patients with this method. Tulp reports excellent results after a follow-up of 7.2 years with resection of the radial head (76%) as compared to 70% without resection of the radial head and as low as 43% when silastic was used.

Activity and duration of participation of the joint probably do not influence the result. In addition to limited function, pain is also an important criterion for indication of surgery [4]. According to Waertel [18] and Wessinghage [36], the form of the disease is decisive for therapy. The authors distinguish between cystic-mutilating and secondary arthrotic forms. However, they recommend synovectomy for treatment of both forms; only in the case of cystic-mutilating disease with increasing instability should implantation of an endoprosthesis be performed.

As a consequence of the multitude of conclusions drawn by several authors, we conclude that in the case of a stable elbow joint, late synovectomy is indicated, taking into consideration the initial situation. This method of surgery results in a long-lasting reduction in pain and in an increase in the range of motion; it renders subsequent surgery such as arthroplasty or implantation of an endoprosthesis only slightly more difficult and therefore enables later performance of more extended surgery.

References

1. Boyle JA, Buchanan WW (1971) Clinical rheumatology. Blackwell Sientific, Oxford
2. Gschwend N (1977) Die operative Behandlung der chronischen Polyarthritis mit einem Beitrag von Albert Böni, 2nd edn. Thieme, Stuttgart
3. Rainer F, Siegmeth W (1985) Handbuch der Inneren Medizin (ed: H Mathies). Springer, Berlin Heidelberg New York
4. Porter BB, Richardson C, Vainio K (1974) Rheumatoid arthritis of the elbow: the results of synovectomy. J Bone Joint Surg 56B:427–437
5. Vojtisek O (1968) Einige klinische Beobachtungen und Laborbefunde mit Rücksicht auf die Frühdianose der primär chronischen Polyarthritis. Beitr Rheumatol 13:21–29
6. Fleming A, Benn RT, Corbett M, Wood PHN (1976) Early rheumatoid disease, part I and II. Ann Rheum Dis 35:357–364

7. Marmor L (1972) Surgery of the rheumatoid elbow – follow-up study on synovectomy combined with radial head excision. J Bone Joint Surg 54A:573–578
8. Tulp NJA, Winia WPCA (1989) Synovectomy of the elbow in rheumatoid arthritis – long term results. J Bone Joint Surg 71B:664–668
9. Larsen A, Dale K, Eek M (1977) Radiographic evaluation of rheumatoid arthritis and related conditions by standard reference films. Acta Radiol 18:481–491
10. Ferlic DC, Clayton EP, Clayton ML, Freeman AC (1987) Elbow synovectomy in rheumatoid arthritis – long-term results. Clin Orthop 220:119–125
11. Vahvanen V, Eskola A, Peltonen J (1991) Results of elbow synovectomy in rheumatoid arthritis. Arch Orthop Trauma Surg 110:151–154
12. Tressel W, Kähler G, Mohing W, Stephan E (1989) Ergebnisse der Synovektomie des Ellbogengelenkes bei chronischer Polyarthritis. Aktuel Probl Chir Orthop 37:57–60
13. Stein H, Dickson RA, Bentley G (1975) Rheumatoid arthritis of the elbow. Pattern of joint involvement, and results of synovectomy with excision of the radial head. Ann Rheum Dis 34:403–408
14. Rymaszewski LA, Mackay I, Amis AA, Miller JH (1975) Long term effects of excision of the radial head in rheumatoid arthritis. J Bone Joint Surg 66B:109–113
15. Brumfield RH, Resnick CT (1985) Synovectomy of the elbow in rheumatoid arthritis. J Bone Joint Surg 67A:16–20
16. Waertel G, Wessinghage D, Zacher J (1989) Differentialindikation, OP-Technik und Nachbehandlungskonzept der Ellbogengelenkseingriffe beim Polyarthritiker. Aktuel Probl Chir Orthop 37:46–54
17. Siekmann W, Beyer W, Hagena FW, Weseloh G, Refior HJ (1989) Einfluß der Radius-köpfchenresektion auf das Ergebnis der Synovectomie des Ellbogengelenkes bei chronischer Polyarhritis. Aktuel Probl Chir Orthop 37:61–64
18. Copeland ṢA, Taylor JG (1979) Synovectomy of the elbow in rheumatoid arthritis – the place of excision of the head of the radius. J Bone Joint Surg 61B:69–73
19. Grimm J (1989) Spätsynovektomie des Ellenbogens und Resektion des Radiusköpfchens bei chronischer Polyarthritis. Z Orthop 127:77–81
20. Eichenblat M, Hass A, Kessler I (1982) Synovectomy of the elbow in rheumatoid arthritis. J Bone Joint Surg 64A:1074–1078
21. Taylor AR, Mukerjea SK, Rana NA (1976) Excision of the head of the radius in rheumatoid arthritis. J Bone Joint Surg 58B:485–487¡
22. Morrey BF, Askew LJ, An KN, Chao EY (1981) A biomechanical study of normal functional elbow motion. J Bone Joint Surg 61A:872–877
23. Inglis AE, Ranawatt CS, Straub LR (1971) Synovectomy and debridement of the elbow in rheumatoid arthritis. J Bone Joint Surg 53A:652–662
24. Saito T, Koshino T, Okamoto R, Horiuchi S (1986) Radical synovectomy with muscle release for rheumatoid elbow. Acta Orthop Scand 57:71–73
25. Wilson DW, Arden GP, Ansell BM (1973) Synovectomy of the elbow in rheumatoid arthritis. J Bone Joint Surg 55B:106–111
26. Linclau LA, Winia WP, Korst JK (1983) Synovectomy of the elbow in rheumatoid arthritis. Acta Orthop Scand 53:935–937
27. Rymaszewski L, Mackay I, Amis A, Miller JH (1984) Long term effects of the excision of the radial head in rheumatold arthritis. J Bone Joint Surg 66B:66–109
28. Gschwend N, Steiger JU (1986) Ellbogengelenk. Orthopäde 15:304–312
29. Weseloh G (1989) Einführung. Aktuel Probl Chir Orthop 37:106–119
30. Torgerson WR, Leach RE (1970) Synovectomy of the elbow in rheumatoid arthritis. J Bone Joint Surg 52A:371–375
31. Böhler N, Czurda R, Schwägerl W, Endler M (1979) Erweiterte Ellenbogen-Synovektomie bei primärer chronischer Polyarthritis. Fortschr Med 27:1179–1184
32. Gschwend N (1980) Surgical treatment of rheumatoid arthritis. Thieme, Stuttgart
33. Keret D, Porter KM (1984) Synovial cyst and ulnar nerve entrapement. Clin Orthop Relat Res 188:213–216

34. Ishikawa H, Hirohata K (1990) Posterior interosseous nerve syndrome associated with rheumatoid synovial cysts of the elbow joint. Clin Orthop Related Res 254:134–139
35. Mackay I, FritzGerald B, Miller JH (1982) Silastic radial head prosthesis in rheumatoid arthritis. Acta Orthop Scand 53:63–66
36. Wessinghage D (1986) Makropathologische Veränderungen bei chronischen Polyarthritiden – Grundlagen einer neuen Phaseneinteilung des Krankheitsverlaufes. Z Orthop 124:437

Resection Interposition Arthroplasty of the Elbow in Rheumatoid Arthritis

W. Rüther and K. Tillmann

Introduction

Resection interposition arthroplasties are well-established procedures in rheumatoid arthritis. They are performed in the forefoot, in the metacarpophalangeal joint, in the shoulder, wrist joint, acromioclavicular joint, and in the elbow joint, among others.

The underlying principles and ideas for resection arthroplasties go back to the last century. Ollier [21] in France is regarded as the first to try to remobilize stiff elbow joints and as early as 1882 he reported on 106 resection arthroplasties. Helferich [8] introduced interposition of muscle flaps to prevent reankylosis. In the following 30 years, important contributions were made by McAusland [18], and Campbell [3] from the United States, by Putti [24] from Italy, and by Payr [22] and Lexer [15] from Germany. Payr (from Greifswald in Germany) proposed resection arthoplasties for many joints. He even recommended resection arthroplasty of the elbow with a distraction device (Fig. 1), which in principles is now being recommended again, e.g., by Morrey [18]. The aim of resection arthroplasties at that time was remobilization of stiff joints. The interposed material therefore was essential to prevent reankylosis. It was Herbert [9] in France and Vainio [33] in Finland who recommended resection arthroplasty not only for stiff joints, but also for destructed, painful elbow joints and rheumatoid joints. Nowadays resection arthroplasties are mainly confined to rheumatoid patients, and it is not stiffness of the joint that is the main indication for surgery, but pain. This is very important in term of the interposed material.

After the introduction of the modern artificial joints, the classical surgical methods, such as osteotomies, arthrodeses, and autoarthroplasties have been gradually forced aside. The question arises whether the classical method of resection arthroplasty still has a role to play in the modern concept of rheumatoid arthritis surgery. This question seems to be of special interest in the elbow. Resection arthroplasties have proved to be most useful in this joint, whereas endoprosthetic replacement of the elbow has so far created many problems.

It is generally accepted that, in early stages of elbow joint involvement in rheumatoid arthritis, synovectomy gives good results, at least in terms of pain relief. Even in more advanced destruction of the elbow, late synovectomies have been recommended. However, if the articular surface is destroyed and deformed

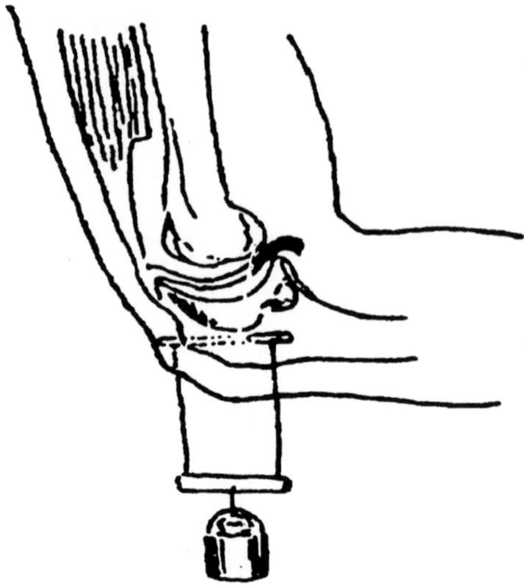

Fig. 1. Resection interposition arthroplasty of the elbow with distraction device of Payr [22]

and prevents congruous motion, either resurfacing by endoprosthetic replacement or recontouring and reshaping by resection arthroplasty is needed [1, 2, 4–6, 10, 16, 20, 23, 25, 29, 31].

Resection arthroplasty has one important advantage: even in destroyed articular surfaces an endoprosthesis is not needed. On the other hand, several factors detract from the popularity of resection arthroplasties in rheumatoid arthritis:

1. The simplification of articular surfaces. From a theoretical standpoint, resection arthroplasties cannot aim at a perfect reconstruction of the surfaces, which may cause continuing pain.
2. A kind of adverse relationship between mobility and stability is suggested.
3. Different amounts of bone resorption are observed in rheumatoid arthritis that may interfer with joint stability.
4. Resection interposition arthroplasty has been suggested to deteriorate with time, either because of secondary osteoarthritis or because of gross bone resorption impairing stability.

These are the four main reasons why the procedure has been judged as unpredicable in its end result.

Surgical Procedure in Rheumatoid Arthritis

In contrast to Ollier [21] and Hass [7] minimal bone resection is preferred. A longitudinal dorsal incision, curving to the radial side of the olecranon, is made. A long reverse V-shaped flap of the triceps aponeurosis is elevated off the underlying muscle. The triangular flap is left attached to the olecranon. After synovectomy, the tips of the olecranon and the coronoid process are smoothed. The radial head is removed from a lateral incision, preserving the anular ligament. The intercondylar bone of the distal humerus is reshaped to a smoothly curved concavity. Finally, the distal humerus is covered by freeze dried dura mater allograft, using three to four drill holes [30].

In cases of ulnar nerve symptoms, the nerve is translocated anteriorly. In rare cases large cysts need to be grafted.

The rehabilitation program is facilitated by using three plaster spints, with the elbow in maximal flexion, maximal extension, and at a right angle. The splints were applied several times a day for several hours. Overnight and for rest the right-angled splint is used.

Patients

From 1969 to 1988, 72 patients with rheumatoid arthritis were treated by resection interposition arthroplasty. By the time the follow-up study had started, 16 patients had died and three were lost to follow-up; 53 patients and 61 joints were reexamined. There were 48 women and five men.

The follow-up time ranged from 1 to 19 years, with a mean of 7.1 years. The patients were divided into three groups: follow-up of less than 5 years (17 joints), follow-up of 5–10 years (32 joints), and follow-up of more than 10 years (12 joints).

Evaluation was performed using a questionaire and by X-ray and clinical examination. Not all the patients underwent each of these evaluations. For this reason, the number of patients differ slightly for each criterium. The exact number for each criterium is given separately in the respective figures and tables.

Indication for surgery in all cases was advanced involvement of the elbow in rheumatoid arthritis with radiographic changes according to Larson stages III–V [14]. The primary indication for surgery in all patients was pain that had not responded to conservative treatment. An increase in the range of motion was not the primary objective of the procedure, but limitation of range of motion constituted a secondary indication.

Mobility

Active flexion and extension improved on average from 70° to 100° (Fig. 2). Stiff joints improved less than mobile joints. In only a few patients was a significant loss of motion observed (Fig. 3). The gain of flexion was preserved over the years, whereas improvement of extension was lost in patients at long-term follow-up (Fig. 4). Regarding forearm rotation, improvement nearly exclusively concerns supination (Fig. 5). After more than 10 years, only a few degrees of this gain remained.

Comparison of patients with different follow-up times indicated that there was a reduction of postoperative improvement at long-term follow-up, particularly regarding extension and supination, which gradually approached the preoperative status. The flexion persisted.

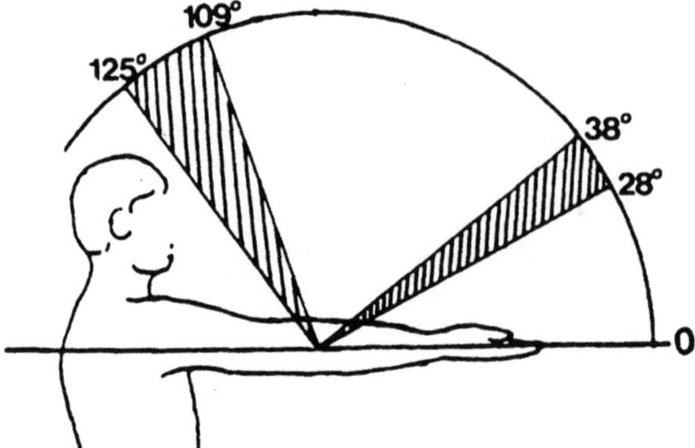

Fig. 2. Flexion and extension in resection interposition arthroplasty before (0°–38°–109°) and after (0°–28°–125°) operation ($n = 57$). Mean follow-up, 7.1 years (range, 1–19 years)

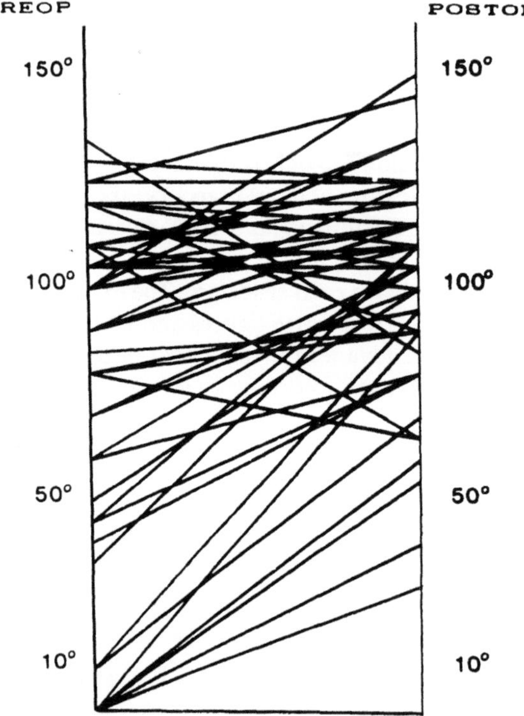

Fig. 3. Gain and loss in range of motion pre- and postoperatively

Stability

Results in joint stability correspond to these observations. Stability was evaluated by passive motion in extension. On average, the joints became more stable with time, probably due to increasing fibrous fixation (Fig. 6). There was no correlation between stability and the amount of bone resorption. It is an important fact that even patients with marked instability e.g., 20°–30° in each direction, were com-

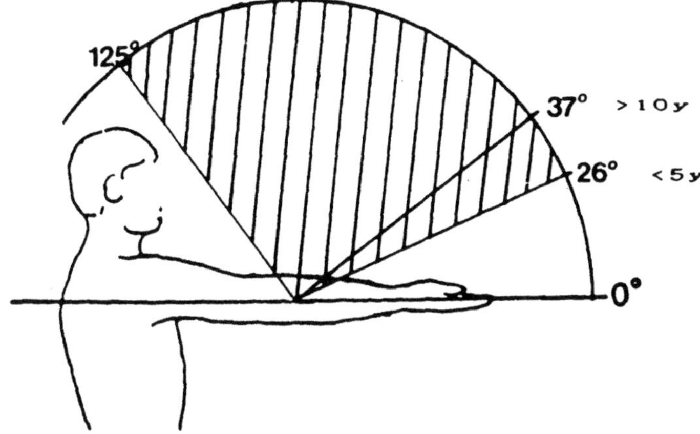

Fig. 4. Loss of extension in the long-term follow-up group (>10 years) compared to the short-term follow-up group (<5 years)

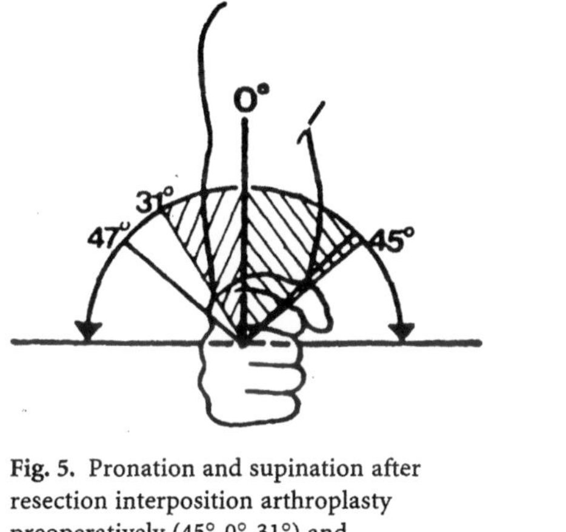

Fig. 5. Pronation and supination after resection interposition arthroplasty preoperatively (45°-0°-31°) and postoperatively (44°-0°-47°)

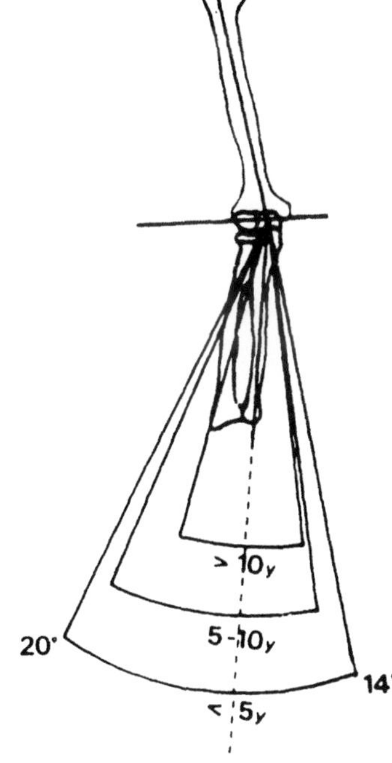

Fig. 6. Improving stability in the different follow-up groups

pletely satisfied, though they sometimes had reservations regarding weight-bearing. No correlation was established between stability and subjective assessment. However, nine patients felt that instability more or less impaired their activities of daily living.

Table 1. Evaluation of pain, no deterioration after time

Degree of pain	Joints		Follow-up (years)		
	(*n*)	(%)	<5	5–10	>10
Severe	4	6.7	3	1	–
Moderate	9	15	2	6	1
Mild	13	21.7	6	2	5
None	34	56.7	9	19	6
Total number of joints	60		20	28	11

Table 2. Patients' assessment of the result of resection interposition arthroplasty

Assessment	Joints	
	(*n*)	(%)
Satisfield	42	69
Satisfied with reservations	7	11
Not satisfied (pain, instability, small range of motion)	12	20
Total number of joints	61	

Pain

Regarding pain, nearly 80% of our patients felt no pain or had pain only after enforced activity (Table 1); 15% needed additional medication because of elbow pain. It must be pointed out, however, that most of the patients were on nonsteroidal anti-inflammatory medication because of multiple joint involvement. Only 7% of the patients had continous pain even at rest. Pain relief showed no deterioration with time. In this respect the operation yielded persisting good results.

In summary, 80% of the patients felt satisfied, and 20% were not satisfied because of pain or instability or were disappointed with joint mobility (Table 2). These 20% of patients include the patients who later underwent revision. Most of them were in to the short-term follow-up group.

Complications

There was a high rate of ulnar nerve complaints, mostly transient deficiencies in sensibility (Table 3). Four patients underwent revision within the first 2 years after resection interposition arthroplasty for translocation of the ulnar nerve.

Table 3. Complications following resection interposition arthroplasty
of the elbow

Complications	Joints	
	(*n*)	(%)
Ulnar never irritation	16	26
Epicondylar/ulnar fracture	5	8
Ectopic ossification	3	7
Infection	–	–
Triceps rupture	–	–
Revisions	9	15
Ulnar never transfers	4	
Endoprosthetic replacements	3	
Osteosynthesis of fracture	2	

There were five fractures of the humeral condyle or the olecranon. One fragment was removed during ulnar nerve revision. Two fractures underwent internal fixation and two were left without symptoms. Ectopic ossifications are mentioned only for the sake of completeness, as they never resulted in significant symptoms.

In three cases, endoprosthetic replacement was performed within the first 2 years because of enduring pain and disappointing mobility. Endoprosthetic replacement was not used for joint instability.

Bone Resorption

It has not yet been determined whether bone resorption should be classified as a short-term or a long-term complication or whether it is an inevitable feature of this procedure in rheumatoid arthritis.

The reactions of bone after resection interposition arthroplasty can be roughly divided into two types: the resorptive and the productive type. The productive type is more frequent in osteoarthritis, e.g. after trauma, and and is a relatively rare condition in rheumatoid arthritis. This type of bony reaction is characterized by early development of osteophytes, joint space narrowing, and bony sclerosis (Fig. 7). This type tends to result in limited mobility. Thus, the results of resection interposition arthroplasty in osteoarthritis, particularly after trauma, should be differentiated from the results in rheumatoid arthritis.

In rheumatoid arthritis, the resorptive type of bony reaction is commonly found, manifesting itself over time in osteolytic changes of the adjacent bones (Fig. 8). If it occurs, bone resorption develops slowly with time. It is not a kind of bony collapse that rapidly causes massive bone loss. Usually, a subtle bone sclerosis develops within the few first weeks after the operation. Bone will subsequently be gradually resorbed (Fig. 9). Sometimes the resorptive activity seems to stop after several months or years. However, even after 10 years or more further bone loss

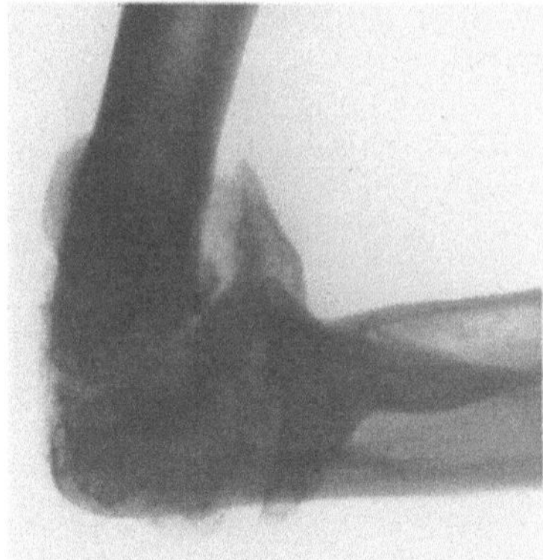

Fig. 7. Productive bone reaction 7 years after resection interposition arthroplasty for post-traumatic osteoarthritis

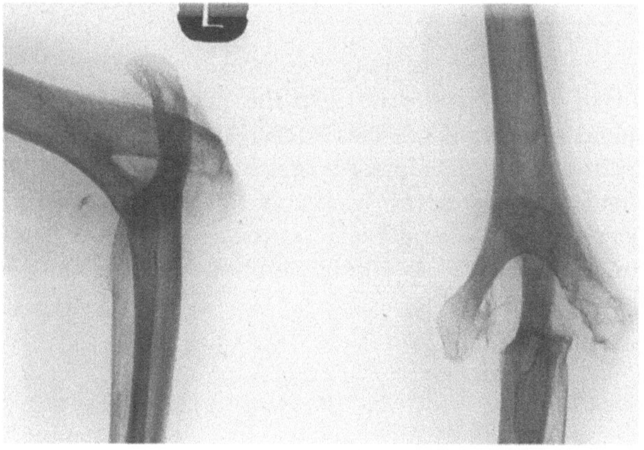

Fig. 8. Massive bone resorption in the intercondylar area, including the fossa olecrani, 12 years after resection interposition arthroplasty in rheumatoid arthritis

can be observed in some cases. Thus it is logical that severe bone resorption is mostly found after 10 years or more.

Nearly 80% of our cases developed bone resorption to a greater or lesser extent (Table 4). Most frequently and most seriously affected is the intercondylar area of the distal humerus. To a lesser extent the semilunar notch and the proximal end of the radius are involved. In 30% of our cases gross bone resorption occurred. Gross bone resorption means a loss of bone that includes the fossa olecrani on X-ray control in the dorsocubital view. There is a predisposition to spontanous condylar fractures in these cases, suggesting pronounced instability [27]. However, there was no correlation between the amount of bone resorption and joint instability if fracture did not occur.

The reasons for bone resorption are not yet fully understood. The following aspects must be taken into consideration.

1. Recurrent synovitis. There may be cases in which recurrent synovitis contributes to bone loss, but in general bone resorption cannot be solely due to recurrent synovitis. Clinical and radiologic signs of recurrence are usually lacking and bone resorption procedes without any pain.

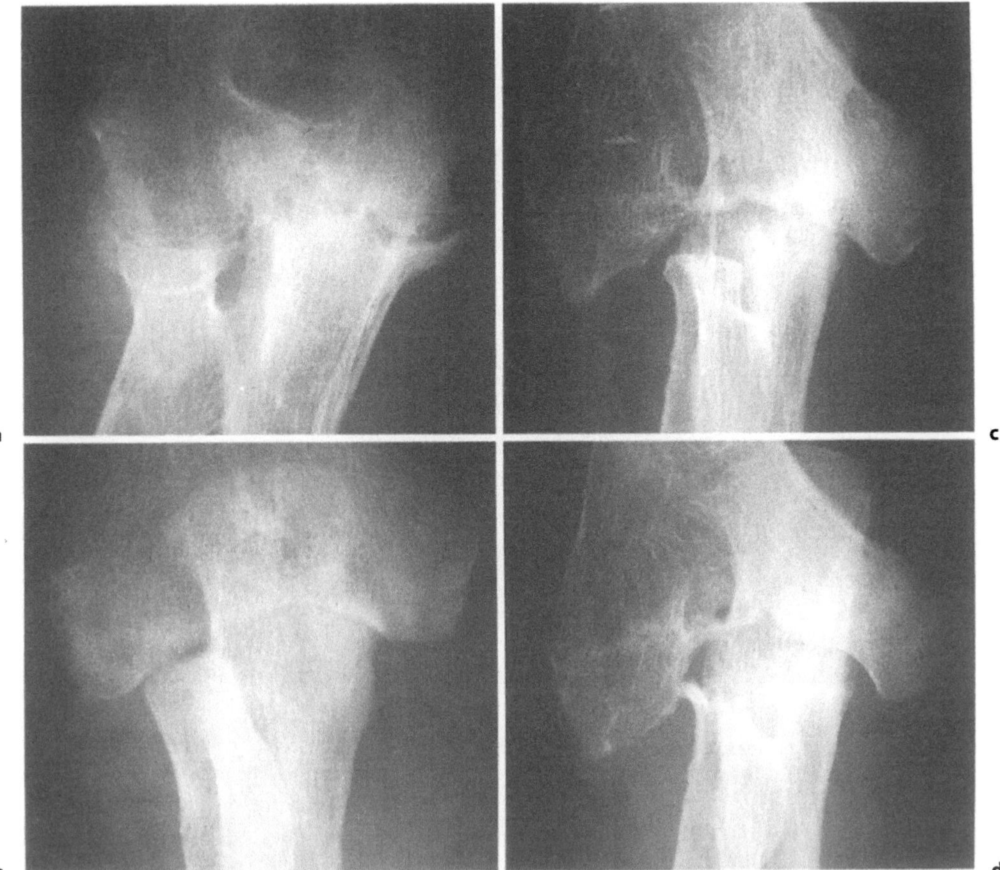

Fig. 9. a Preoperative X-ray. b Four weeks after arthroplasty, subtle bone sclerosis in the intercondylar area. c Minor bone resorption in the intercondylar area 2 years after arthroplasty. d Moderate bone resorption 5 years after arthroplasty, nearly reaching the fossa olecrani

Table 4. Bone resorption in the distal humerus

Extent of resorption	Joints	
	(n)	(%)
No resorption	10	22
Minor resorption	13	29
Resorption, reaching fossa olecrani	8	18
Resorption, including fossa olecrani	14	31
Total number of joints	45	100

2. Drug therapy. The influence of anti-inflammatory drugs on osteoblastic activity may be of importance, e.g., indometacine, cortisone, and methotrexate.
3. Mutilation. There is probably is a disease-dependent factor that varies individually and that causes predisposition to bone resorption and mutilation. In this respect, the spontanous changes in other joints can, with some reservations, be used to predict the development of severe resorption after resection interposition arthroplasty.
4. Interposition material. The significance of the implanted freeze-dried dura mater membrane is still unknown. Bone resorption has been observed in other kinds of arthroplasty of the elbow joint [11, 13, 17, 26, 28, 32–34]. Furthermore, it is not known whether there are differences related to the surgical technique.
5. Mechanical factors. On the basis of the above-mentioned factors, mechanical factors must be taken into consideration. They probably play a major role in modeling the new shape of articulating surfaces [6].

Conclusions

In summary, we feel resection interposition arthroplasty to be a reliable procedure in advanced elbow involvement in rheumatoid arthritis, particular in young patients. Results do not deteriorate with time, neither regarding pain nor mobility nor stability. The limited bone resection does not imply joint stiffness, as suggested in osteoarthritis. On the other hand, limited bone resection does not prevent gross bone resorption in all cases. If there is preexisting severe instability, endoprosthetic replacement may be preferred. Mutilation types of cases should be excluded from this procedure, and in stiff joints a distraction device may be considered.

In many cases there is no need to implant an endoprosthesis and to merely regard resection arthroplasty as a possible salvage procedure. In our hands resection interposition arthroplasty remains an excellent first option in carefully selected individuals and endoprosthetic replacement may be the salvage procedure, if necessary. However, with growing confidence in the endoprosthetic replacement of the elbow, this therapeutic concept will probably need revision.

References

1. Bontemps G, Meier G, Tillmann K (1975) Synovektomie und Arthroplastiken des Ellenbogengelenkes bei chronischer Polyarthritis. Orthop Prax 11:895–899
2. Brumfield RH, Resnick CT (1985) Synovectomy of the elbow in rheumatoid arthritis. J Bone Joint Surg 67A:16–20
3. Campbell WC (1922) Arthroplasty of the elbow. Ann Surg 76:615
4. Dickson RA, Stein H, Bentley G (1976) Excision arthroplasty of the elbow in rheumatoid disease. J Bone Joint Surg 58B:227–228
5. Ferlic DC, Patchett CE, Clayton ML, Freeman AC (1987) Elbow synovectomy in rheumatoid arthritis. Clin Orthop 220:119–125

6. Gschwend N (1977) Die operative Behandlung der chronischen Polyarthritis. Thieme, Stuttgart, pp 63–68

7. Hass J (1930) Die Mobilisierung ankylotischer Ellenbogen- und Kneiegelenke mittels Arthroplastik. Langenbecks Arch Klin Chir 160:693–715

8. Helferich H (1894) Ein neues Operationsverfahren zur Heilung der Knöchernen Kiefergelenksankylose. Verh Dtsch Ges Chir 23:504–510

9. Herbert JJ (1958) Traitement des ankyloses du coude dans le rheumatisme. Rev Chir Orthop 44:87

10. Inglis AE (1985) Rheumatoid arthritis. In: Morrey BF (ed) The elbow and its disorders. Saunders, Philadelphia, pp 638–655

11. Kimura C, Vainio K (1976) Arthroplasty of the elbow. Arch Orthop Unfallchir 84:339-348

12. Knight RA, Van Zandt IL (1952) Arthroplasty of the elbow: an end result study. J Bone Joint Surg 36A:610

13. Koneczny O, Marx C, von Leeuwen P (1985) Die Korium-Interpositionsplastik des Ellenbogen- und Handgelenkes. Handchirurgie 17:18–22

14. Larsen A, Dale K, Eek M (1977) Radiographic evaluation of rheumatoid arthritis and related conditions by standard reference films. Acta Radiol 18:481–491

15. Lexer E (1909) Über Gelenktransplantationen. Arch Klin Chir 90:263

16. Linclau LA, Winia WPCA, von der Korst JK (1983) Synovectomy of the elbow in rheumatoid arthritis. Acta Orthop Scand 54:935–937

17. Matsuno S, Ishii S, Minami M (1985) Arthroplasty of the elbow joint with the OMS's membrane. In: Kashiwagi D (ed) Elbow joint. Excerpta Medica, Amsterdam, pp 249–254

18. McAusland WR (1947) Arthroplasty of the elbow. N Engl J Med 236:97–99

19. Morrey BF (1994) Distraction arthroplasty. In: Morrey BF (ed) The elbow. Raven New York, pp 307–328

20. Neumann R (1986) Die Interpositionsarthroplastik am Ellenbogengelenk bei der chronischen Polyarthritis. Z Rheumatol 45:208–209

21. Ollier (1882) Demonstration anatomique de la reconstitution du coude après la resection sousperiostee. Examen d'une série de 106 cas de cette operation. Zentralbl Chir 9:548–549

22. Payr E (1910) Über die operative Mobilisierung ankylosierter Gelenke. Munch Med Wochenschr 57:1921–1927

23. Porter BB, Richardson C, Vainio K (1974) Rheumatoid arthritis of the elbow: the results of synovectomy. J Bone Joint Surg 56B:427–437

24. Putti V (1921) Arthroplasty. Am J Orthop Surg 3:421

25. Raunio P, Jakob R (1973) Die Ellenbogenarthroplastik in der rheumatoiden Arthritis. Orthopade 2:102–104

26. Shahriaree H, Sajadi K, Silver CM, Sheikholeslamza S (1979) Excisional arthroplasty of the elbow. J Bone Joint Surg 61A:922–927

27. Sinn W, Hansens C, Tillmann K (1988) Revisionsoperationen am Ellenbogengelenk bei chronischer Polyarthritis. Aktuel Rheumatol 13:183–187

28. Tajima T (1985) Arthroplasty of the elbow joint with J-K membrane. In: Kashiwagi D (ed) Elbow joint. Excerpta Medica, Amsterdam, pp 243–248

29. Thabe H, Tillmann K (1982) Ergebnisse nach Synovektomien des Ellenbogengelenkes. Aktuel Rheumatol 7:1–3

30. Tillmann K (1989) Resektions-Interpositions-Arthroplastik des Ellenbogengelenkes bei chronischer Polyarthritis – Indikation und Ergebnisse. In: Wessinghage D (ed) Das rheumatische Ellenbogengelenk Aktuel Probl Orthop Chir 37:55–56

31. Tillmann K (1990) Recent advances in the surgical treatment of rheumatoid arthritis. Clin Orthop 258:62–72

32. Tsuge K, Murakamu T, Yasunage Y, Kanaujia R (1987) Arthroplasty of the elbow. J Bone Joint Surg 69B:116–120

33. Vainio K (1967) Arthroplasty of the elbow and hand in rheumatoid arthritis. In: Chapchal G (ed) Synovectomy and arthroplasty in rheumatoid arthritis. Thieme, Stuttart, pp 66–70

34. Wright PE, Steward MJ (1985) Fascial arthroplasty of the elbow. In: Morrey B (ed) The elbow and its disorders. Saunders, Philadelphia, pp 530–540

Distraction Arthroplasty of the Elbow

S.W. O'Driscoll and B.F. Morrey

Introduction

Distraction arthroplasty of the elbow was initially described by Volkov and Oganesian in 1975 [1]. Their technique was based on some of Ilizarov's principles of fine-wire external fixation recently popularized in Europe and North America. Deland et al. [2] reported their experience with a hinged external fixation device for the elbow in 1983. Morrey designed a relatively simple hinged external fixation device for distraction arthroplasty of the elbow and has used it since 1986 [3–6]. The kinematics of the normal elbow, which behaves as almost a pure hinge joint in flexion/extension, makes the use of a hinged distractor possible [2, 7–10]. The loci of instant centers of rotation of the elbow for flexion and extension fall within a circle less than 4 mm in diameter. This allows a simple hinged device to be applied to the elbow and the axis of rotation to be simulated by a pin.

Indications

The clear and distinct value of the distraction device is to allow, simultaneous joint motion while ensuring stability by protecting the collateral ligaments. As such, several clinical indications have been recognized in both reconstructive and traumatic surgery.

In reconstructive surgery of the elbow, the most common indication for distraction arthroplasty is post-traumatic stiffness. Though most stiff elbows can be treated without the use of a distractor, the application of a hinged distraction device is generally indicated if 50% or more of the joint surface is void of articular cartilage [11] or if the pathology has modified the joint contour requiring re-fashioning in the joint surface with or without an interposition membrane. The distractor may also be used to stabilize the joint if collateral ligament release was required during surgery.

For traumatic conditions, the distraction device may be applied after unstable dislocations when ligament healing is required. Articular fractures may be protected (unloaded) after fixation by separating the joint while still allowing motion.

Contraindications to the application of this device include local sepsis and the presence of fracture fixation devices in the distal humerus or proximal ulna. The device is also unnecessary after simple capsular release. If the collateral ligaments are intact and the joint surface reasonably normal, there is no need for the distraction device.

Technique

The elbow is exposed according to the pathology present (Fig. 1). If a scar from a previous operation is present, that scar is used or incorporated into the incision whenever possible. Once the deep structures have been exposed, Kocher's interval is entered [12]. Typically the triceps is reflected from the tip of the olecranon, but in some instances, such as when elbow flexion is normal, the triceps may be left intact.

The anterior capsular is excised after exposing it by releasing the common extensor tendon. If the joint surface is intact, the anterior capsular is excised but the lateral collateral ligament is preserved. If the joint is badly damaged, it must be reshaped; the lateral collateral ligament is carefully outlined and elevated as a flap of tissue from the origin at the lateral condyle. This is tagged and reflected distally to provide extensile exposure. A small portion of the proximal tip of the olecranon is removed, and complete anterior and posterior capulectomies are performed. In

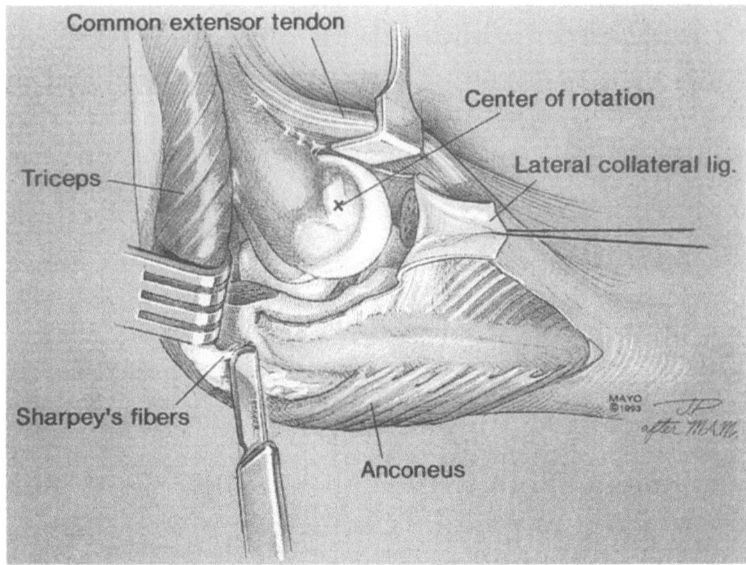

Fig. 1. Surgical approach for distraction arthroplasty. The triceps is reflected in continuity in those instances in which the joint is extremely stiff or when it is anticipated that removal of the collateral ligament will be required. The lateral collateral ligament is elevated from the lateral epicondyle. The lateral margin of the triceps is also elevated from the tip of the olecranon. The center of the axis of rotation of the elbow passes through the lateral epicondyle (*x*). (Reproduced with permission from Mayo Foundation)

instances in which the joint surface is destroyed and must be refashioned, some form of an interposition arthroplasty may be carried out.

The ulnar nerve must be identified, but it may or may not be translocated anteriorly. This is accomplished through the same or a supplemental medial incision, depending on the status of the skin. If a prevous posterior incision is present, a subcutaneous dissection is easily carried out to the medial aspect of the triceps. Protection of the nerve is required at three times during the operation: first during reflection of the triceps, then at the time of capsular dissection, and finally at the time of pin placement for the distraction device. If ulnar nerve symptoms are present before surgery, then the nerve is transposed.

Following exposure of the elbow, the essential landmarks of the distal humerus are identified. On the lateral aspect of the capitellum, a tubercle is present at the site of the origin of the lateral collateral ligament. This tubercle also represents the geometric center of curvature of the capitellum, which is the site of the flexion axis and is the point through which the humeral pin must pass [13]. If this anatomic feature has been altered by pathology, then the center of curvature of the trochlea is identified as the axis of rotation (Fig. 2).

When viewed from the medial side of the distal humerus, the axis of rotation lies just anterior and inferior to the medial epicondyle (Fig. 3). The ulnar nerve is always identified and protected at the time of insertion of the humeral pin. If there is any question with regard to the ulnar nerve, then the pin is inserted from medial to lateral. However, if adequate exposure for accurate placement is present, then we prefer to insert the humeral pin from lateral to medial.

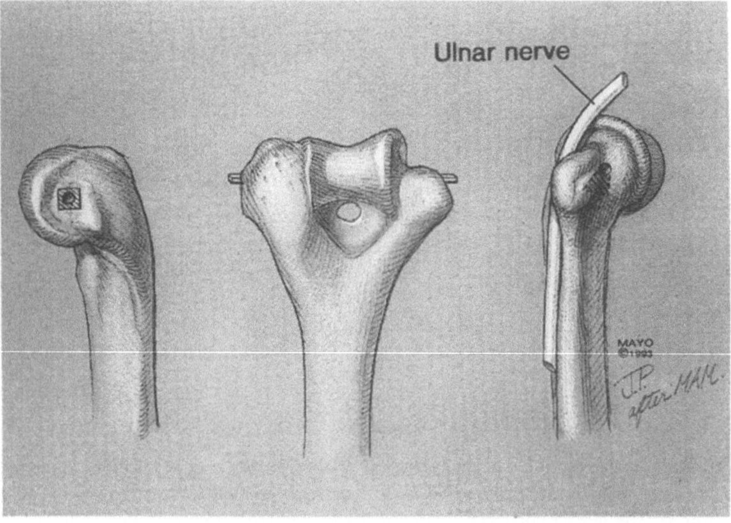

Fig. 2. Landmarks for inserting the distraction device include the lateral epicondyle and the anterior inferior aspect of the medial epicondyle. The axis of rotation of the elbow passes through these two points. (Reproduced with permission from Mayo Foundation)

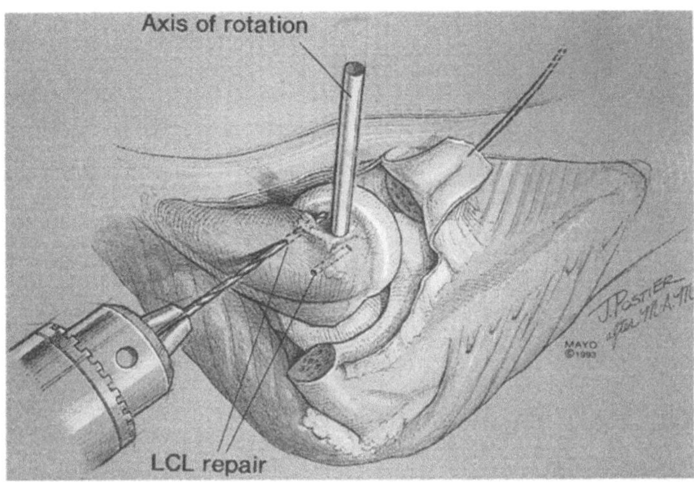

Fig. 3. A drill bit serves both to confirm the orientation of the flexion pin as well as to protect the placement of drill holes for the attachment of the collateral ligaments. (Reproduced with permission from Mayo Foundation)

The exact placement of the pin for the axis of rotation is optimally accomplished by first placing a drill bit across the distal humerus according to the landmarks mentioned above (Fig. 3). A radiograph is taken to assure proper position of the drill bit. The drill bit is removed and a 4-mm threaded Steinmann pin is then driven across the distal humerus. First, the skin is punctured laterally, taking care to ensure that the incision is far enough anterior so as to allow skin closure without being under tension. The emergence of the flexion pin is observed medially while the ulnar nerve is being protected. The anterior skin flap is drawn posteriorly and the threaded pin is allowed to puncture the skin medially.

After placement of the humeral pin, two smooth pins are then placed in the ulna posterior and anterior to the center of the articulation in the regions of the olecranon and approximately 5 cm distally in the ulna (Fig. 4). These pins are also placed percutaneously, but this portion of the ulna has usually been exposed so it is not difficult to identify and execute the proper insertion site of these pins. Both pins should be placed parallel to each other and parallel to the humeral pin as viewed in both the anteroposterior (AP) and the lateral plane (Fig. 5).

The lateral collateral ligament is then secured, as is the common extensor tendon (Fig. 6). If the triceps has been reflected, this is then reattached with the suture placed prior to the pins being inserted (Figs. 6, 7).

The distraction of the ulna is accomplished by advancing the distraction device. Typically, approximately 3–5 mm of distraction of the joint surface is desired (Fig. 5). Flexion and extension are assessed and an arc of 40°–110° or more is expected. This should be smooth and no sense of surface contact should be present.

When the elbow is unstable from collateral ligament incompetence or articular incongruity, distraction is a technique that can compensate for such instability.

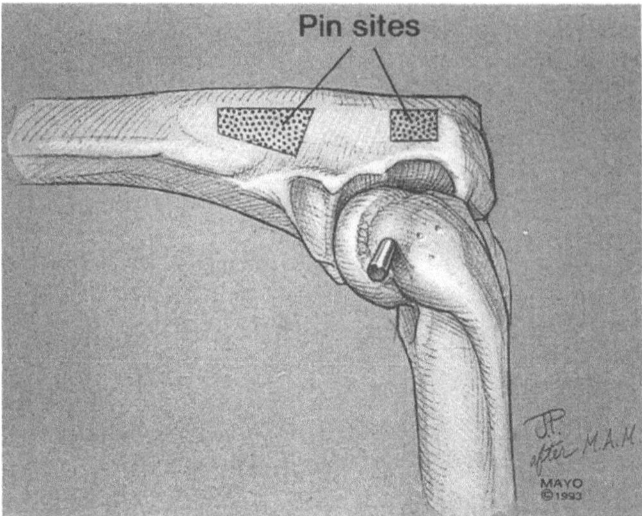

Fig. 4. The insertion sites for the ulnar pins consist of one area in the olecranon region and the other just distal to the coronoid of the proximal ulna. (Reproduced with permission from Mayo Foundation)

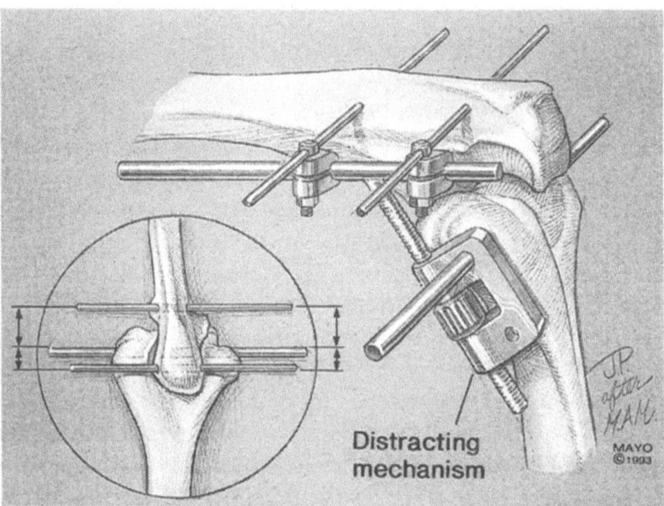

Fig. 5. The ulnar pins are placed parallel to the humeral pin and to each other. The distractor allows distraction of the forearm from the humerus along the line of direction of the collateral ligaments. The ulna is distracted from the humerus 3–5 mm depending upon the circumstances. (Reproduced with permission from Mayo Foundation)

For some acute or subacute fractures, the tendency for posterior subluxation of the ulna may be neutralized by the application of the distraction device (Fig. 8a, b). In this instance the desire is to create an axial distraction along the long axis of the ulna.

The typical features of the application for trauma include: (a) the use of a fluoroscopy so that the pins may be inserted percutaneously, (b) insertion of the

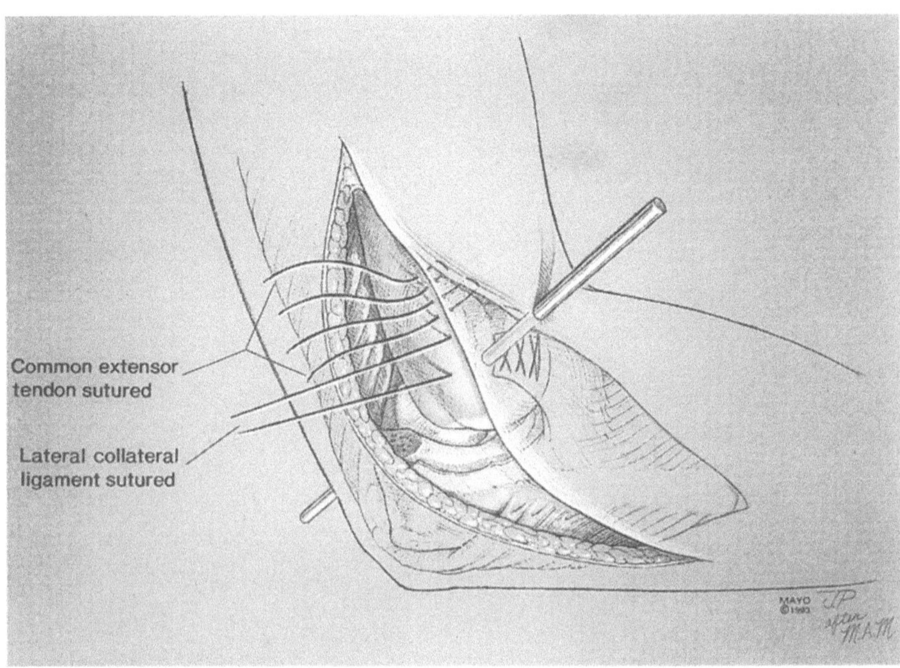

Fig. 6. The humeral flexion pin is placed percutaneously through the skin and then down the channel created by the drill bit. Sutures have been placed in the lateral collateral ligament and the common extensor tendon. (Reproduced with permission from Mayo Foundation)

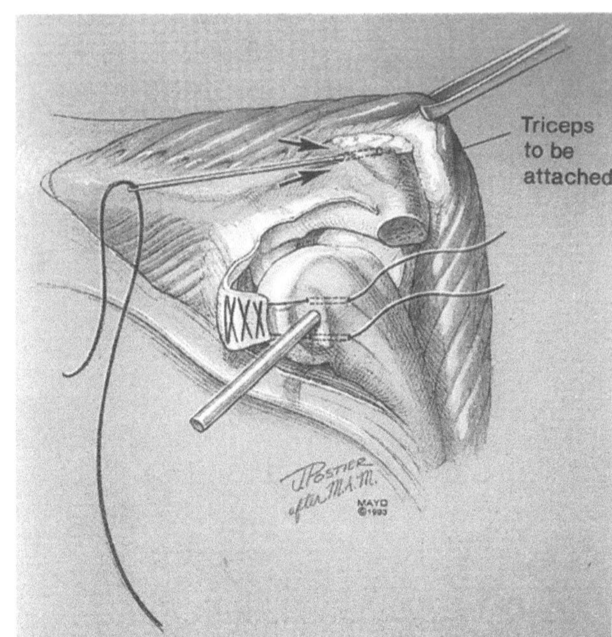

Fig. 7. The collateral ligaments are reattached to the the epicondyles with sutures through drill holes, and the triceps reattached to the olecranon with heavy, nonabsorbable sutures through drill holes. (Reproduced with permission from Mayo Foundation)

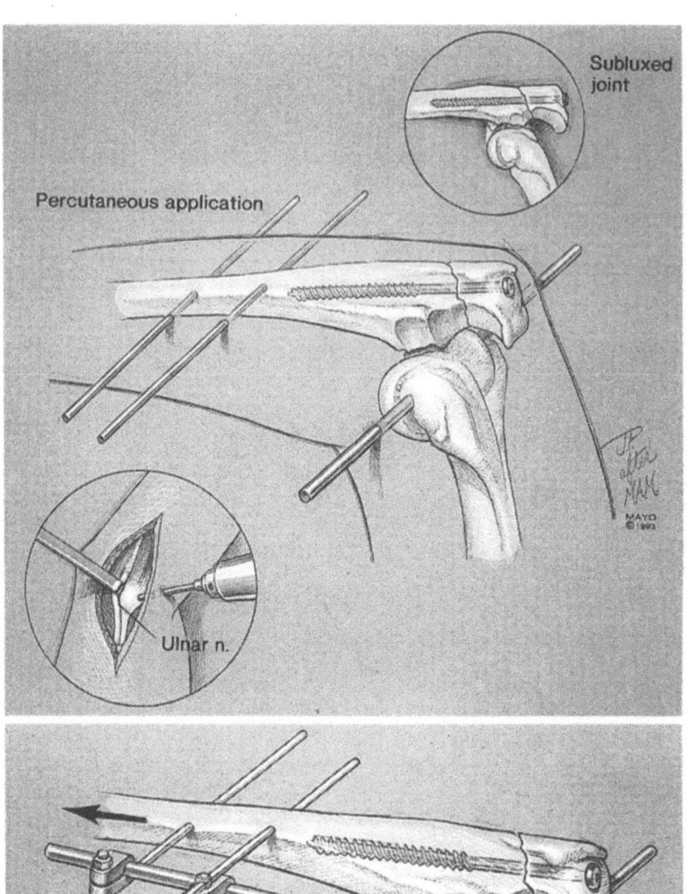

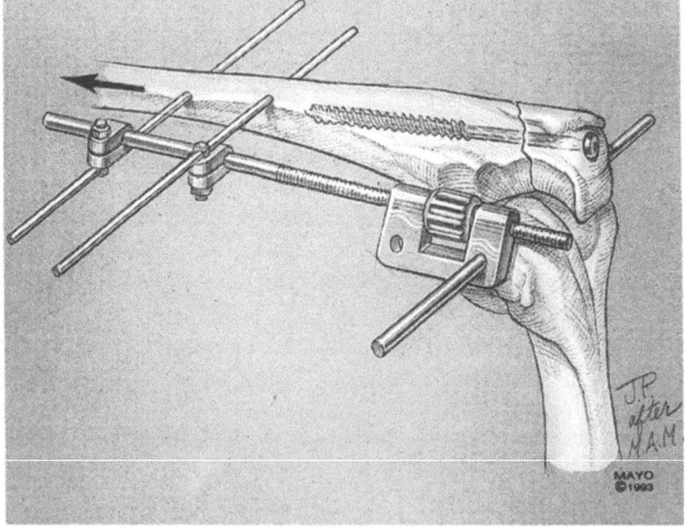

Fig. 8. a The distractor can be used for unstable fracture/dislocations such as coronoid fractures. The ulnar nerve must be identified and protected. **b** An extended device is sometimes used to distract the ulna distally and prevent posterior subluxation of the ulnohumeral joint. (Reproduced with permission from Mayo Foundation)

pins distal to the coronoid to avoid fracture fixation, but also to apply the correct distal displacement vector to accomplish elbow joint reduction, and (c) the use of different type of distraction attachment (Fig. 8).

The ulnar nerve is found with a 3- to 4-cm incision made over the medial epicondyle. The ulnar nerve is simply identified and retracted; it is not translocated. The humeral pin is inserted medially under direct vision with a drill guide in order to avoid any injury to the ulnar nerve and is directed toward the point identified at the lateral condyle. After this pin has been placed, the first ulnar pin is directed through the midportion of the medullary canal of the ulna and distal to any ulnar fracture fixation device. If Steinmann pins or K-wires have been used, as in a tension band wiring technique, the ulna distraction pins may be placed more proximally through the ulna as they will displace the intramedullary pins. The distraction device is then applied using the specific attachment designed for this purpose. The elbow is manually reduced if this is possible. If not, the distraction device is used to assist in the reduction of the elbow. Motion is verified with fluoroscopy.

The third indication is that of the unstable elbow. In this setting the distraction device may be applied, after the elbow has been reduced, as a means of protecting the reconstruction. In the acute setting the percutaneous application described above has been helpful in both reducing the ulnohumeral joint and protecting the reduction, fracture fragments, and collateral ligaments.

Postoperative Management

For most circumstances, we typically employ the following steps postoperatively:

1. Assess the patient in the recovery room to ensure neurovascular competence.
2. A brachial plexus block is accomplished with a local anesthetic using a continuous infusion technique for 2–3 days [14].
3. The extremity is placed in a continuous passive motion (CPM) machine for 4–5 days and the maximum amount of flexion and extension possible with the distraction device is realized within the first 24–48 h [12].
4. If there is no evidence of infection and there has been adequate progress, the patient is dismissed with a portable CPM unit about 5–6 days after surgery.
5. The patient is also allowed unrestricted active motion of the elbow with the distractor in place (Fig. 9).

Approximately 3–4 weeks postoperatively the distraction device is removed and the elbow examined (sometimes under general anesthesia). Care is taken not to formally manipulate the elbow, but some sense of the firmness of the end points of motion is determined since this is felt to have prognostic value.

Anteroposterior and lateral radiographs are taken to ensure that the elbow is adequately reduced and stable (Fig. 10). The patient is then treated with flexion and extension splints, usually for 6–12 weeks after surgery. An additional 3 months of a maintenance program is used to avoid recurrence of the contracture.

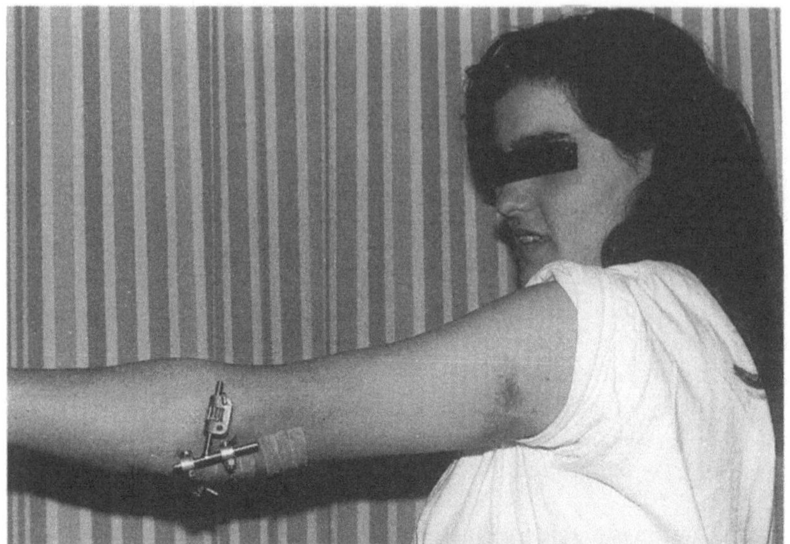

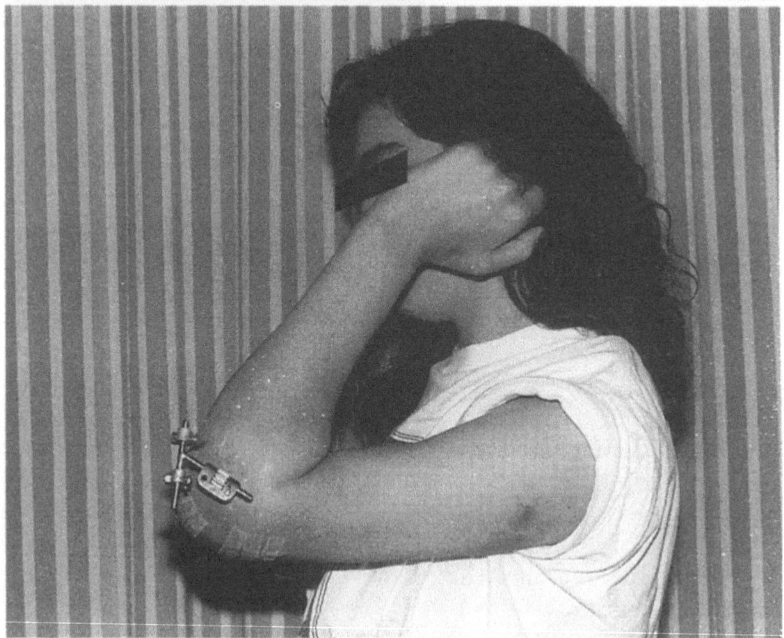

Fig. 9a,b. Clinical photographs of a 22-year-old woman 3 weeks following a distraction arthroplasty of the elbow in which periosteum was used for "biologic resurfacing" of her damaged elbow joint. She had sustained an open fracture/dislocation of the elbow 4 months previously, with disruption of the brachial artery and loss of a large osteochondral fragment of the trochlea and capitellum. Her preoperative motion was from 35° to 110°; at this time 3 weeks postoperatively, her motion was from 20° to 130°. (Reproduced with permission from [15])

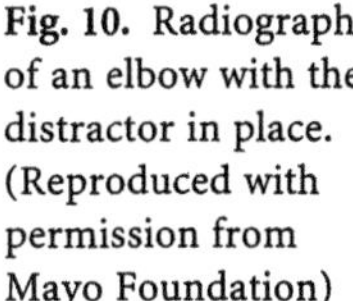

Fig. 10. Radiograph of an elbow with the distractor in place. (Reproduced with permission from Mayo Foundation)

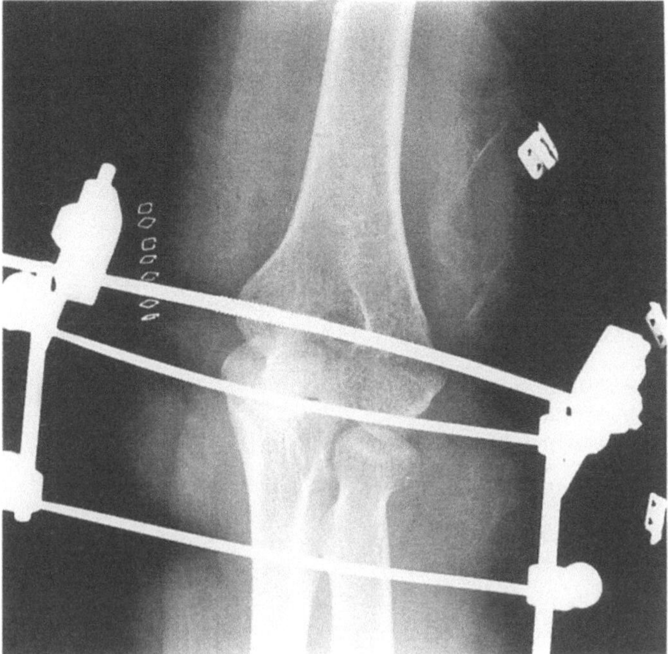

Results

Morrey reported his results of distraction arthroplasty with and without fascia lata interposition for patients in 1990 [6]. In 14 patients who underwent distraction arthroplasty without interposition, their elbow motion improved from a mean arc of 32° preoperatively to 99° postoperatively. A second group of six patients were managed by distraction with fascia lata interposition, and these patients improved from a mean arc of 27° preoperatively to 107° postoperatively. In both groups of patients the arcs of elbow flexion extension were within the functional arc of motion from 30° to 130°.

The device has been used in approximately ten cases of unstable fractures. More than 2 years' follow-up is present in seven cases. Six of these seven have objective scores demonstrating a satisfactory result. One elbow shows residual subluxations.

Complications

Complications of distraction arthroplasty for treating elbow stiffness are frequent, occurring in almost 30% of cases, though most do not affect the long-term outcome and only about 10% require a reoperation (Table 1). The commonest complications are pin site infections and ulnar nerve problems. The distractor sometimes

Table 1. Complications after 64 distraction procedures for elbow stiffness

	No. of cases	Reoperation (*n*)
Infection		
Deep	2	2
Pin site	4	1
Neural		
Ulnar neuritis (temporary)	5	2
Radial neuritis	2	–
Median nerve transection	1	1
Motion lost	1	–
Wound slough (superficial)	1	–
Neurotrophic joint (?)	1	–
Triceps avulsion	1	1
Total	18	7

has to be removed because of infection and persistent drainage. After taking into consideration the complications and reoperations, the overall results are satisfactory in about 90% of cases.

References

1. Volkov MV, Oganesian OV (1975) Restoration of function in the knee and elbow with a hinge distractor. J Bone Joint Surg 57A:591–600
2. Deland JT, Walker PS, Sledge CB, Farberov A (1983) Treatment of posttraumatic elbows with a new hinge-distractor. Orthopaedics 6:732–737
3. Morrey BF (1994) Distraction arthroplasty. In: Morrey BF (ed) Master techniques in orthopedic surgery: the elbow. Raven, New York, pp 307–327
4. Morrey BF (1993) Distraction arthroplasty. Clin Orthop. 293:46–54
5. Morrey BF (1992) Post-traumatic stiffness: distraction arthroplasty. Orthopaedics 15:863–869
6. Morrey BF (1990) Post-traumatic contracture of the elbow. Operative treatment, including distraction arthroplasty. J Bone Joint Surg 72-A:601–618
7. Morrey BF, Chao EY (1976) Passive motion of the elbow joint. A biomechanical analysis. J Bone Joint Surg 58-A:501–508
8. Morrey BF, Askew LJ, An K, Chao EY (1981) A biomechanical study of normal elbow motion. J Bone Joint Surg 63-A:872–877
9. Morrey BF, An K (1983) Articular and ligamentous contributions to the stability of the elbow joint. Am J Sports Med 11:315–319
10. Morrey BF, An K (1985) Functional anatomy of the ligaments of the elbow. Clin Orthop 201:84–90
11. Morrey BF (1990) Treatment of the post-traumatic stiff elbow including distraction arthoplasty. J Bone Joint Surg 72A:601–619
12. Salter RB, Hamilton HW, Wedge JH, Tile M, Torode IP, O'Driscoll SW, Murnaghan JJ, Saringer JH (1984) Clinical application of basic research on continuous passive motion for disorders and injuries of synovial joints: a preliminary report of a feasibility study. J Orthop Res 1:325–342
13. London JT (1981) Kinematics of the elbow. J Bone Joint Surg 63-A:529–535

14. Gaumann DM, Lennon RL, Wedel DJ (1988) Continuous axillary block for postoperative pain management. Reg Anaesth 13:77–81
15. O'Driscoll SW (1993) Surgery of elbow arthritis. In: McCarty DJ, Koopman WJ (eds) Arthritis and allied condition. Lea and Febinger, Philadelphia, pp 951–962

Alloarthroplasty of the Elbow

GSB III Elbow

N. Gschwend, H. Scheier, A. Bähler, and B. Simmen

Introduction

The history of elbow arthroplasty begins in the last century. The procedure of resection arthroplasty started to gain in importance in 1878 when Ollier [1] began to practice it with considerable success. In the 1960s we also used a modification of it in a great number of cases, and we were even able to mobilize elbows which, due to juvenile arthritis, had been ankylosed in extension (Fig. 1). Thirty years after elbow resection arthroplasty, one of these patients is able to use both formerly ankylosed and useless elbows so well that she is independent, can look after herself, and is even able to use two crutches for walking with her multiple joint replacements at the lower extremity.

The main problem of all resection arthroplasties, however, was and still is the reversed relationship between stability and mobility and hence the lack of predictability of when and to what degree the elbow starts to become painful because of instability. In the patient shown in Fig. 1, this phenomenon is convincingly demonstrated: one elbow remained very stable and painless after 30 years, whereas the other one became unstable due to bone resorption and is causing pain. An analysis of a series of 27 patients operated on in the 1960s with a modified resection arthroplasty (method of Hass [2]) demonstrated that one third of all the cases developed painful instability within the first 5 years [3].

No wonder that, based on the very positive experiences made with cemented artificial joints, initially in the hip joint, several authors tried to use the same principle for nonfunctional elbow joints as well. These artificial joints, which were introduced by different authors in the early 1970s, were mainly rigid metal to metal hinges. The exaggerated optimism about this new method is reflected by the fact that most authors deliberately resected both humeral condyles and, with them, the origin of the collateral ligaments before implantation of the artificial joint. An example of this type of prosthesis was the Dee I prosthesis, which inevitably led to severe loosening within the first few years after implantation. Surgeons performing the revision were faced with almost insurmountable difficulties when trying to convert the artificial elbow into a sine – sine (no interpositional material) resection arthroplasty.

In 1971, based on such experiences, Gschwend – together with Scheier and Bähler – decided to construct the GSB I elbow prosthesis, a metal-to-metal hinge

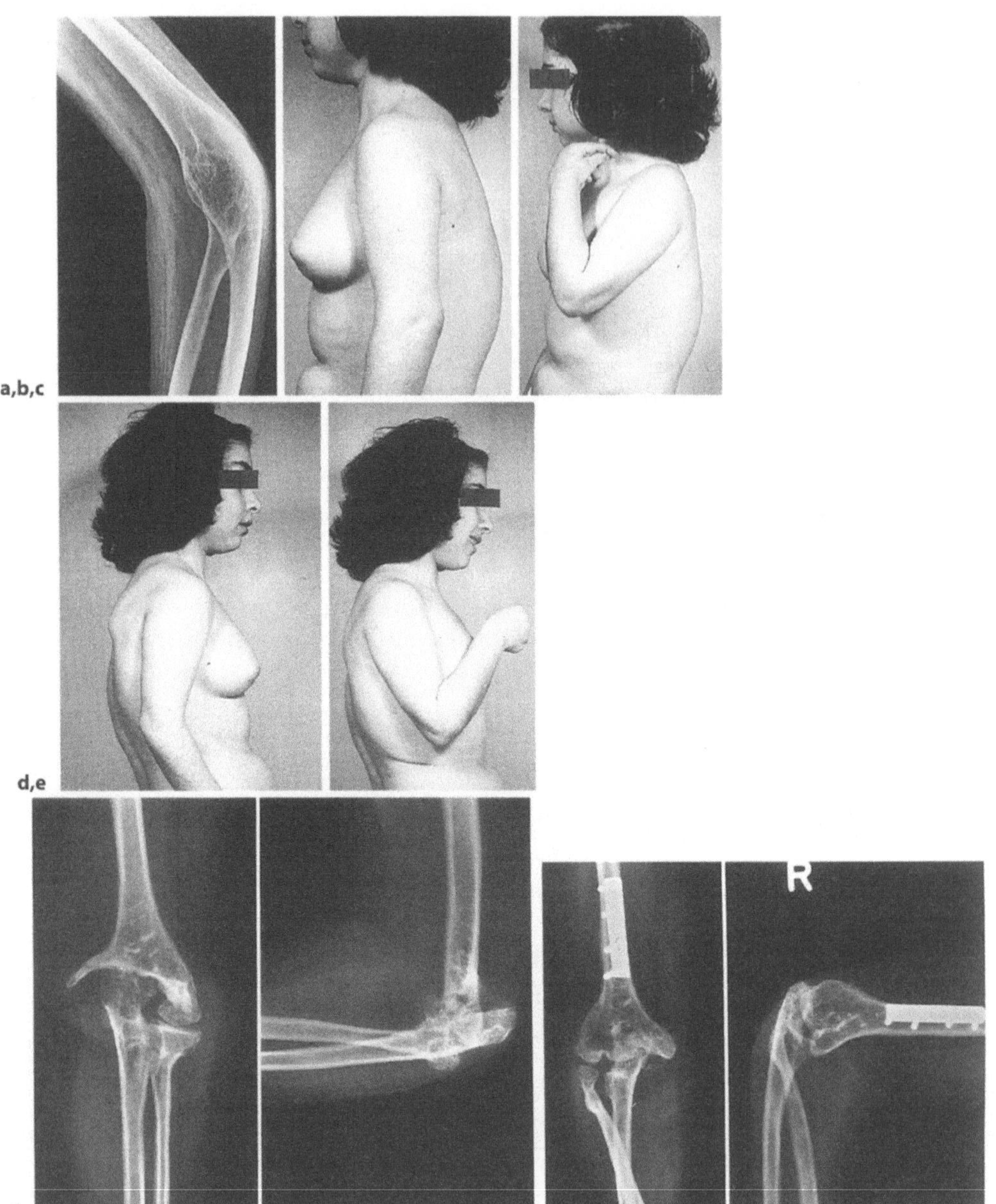

Fig. 1a–e. Bilateral bony ankylosis of both elbows due to juvenile arthritis. Patient unable to be independent. Excellent mobility after bilateral resection arthroplasty. **f,g** Due to bone resorption one elbow became flail and is painful, while the other (*R*) is still very stable and nearly painless

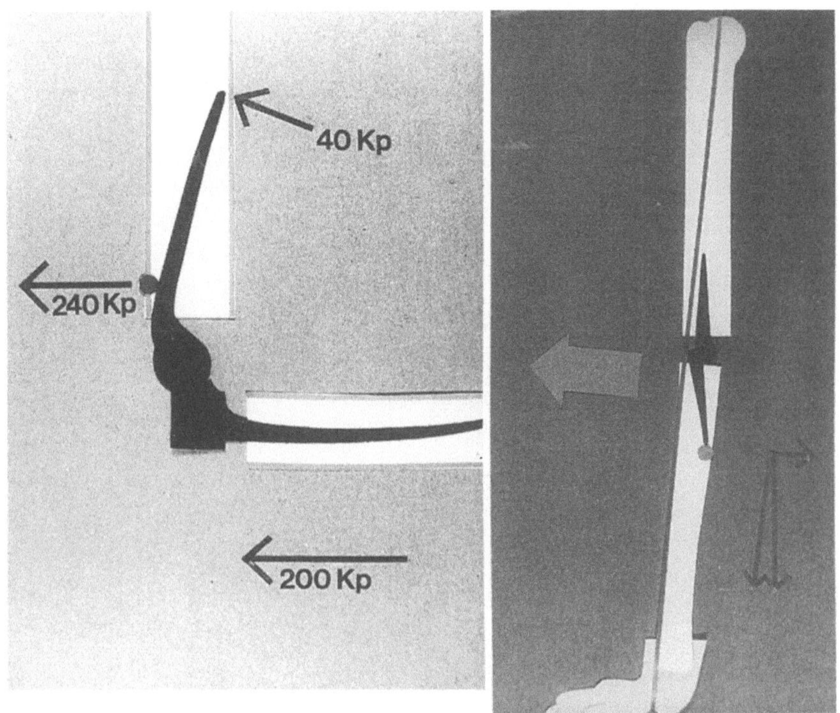

Fig. 2. a Vertical stresses favor subsidence of the humeral component and loosening. **b** When lifting a weight with the elbow flexed, the resultant force works nearly parallel to the ulna (where aseptic loosening only exceptionally happens), but vertically to the posterior wall of the humerus, trying to push the humeral component backwards

joint. In comparison to the above-mentioned method, the advantage of this type of prosthesis was the minimal bone resection necessary between the two humeral condyles for implantation, leaving the ligamentous and muscular origins intact. The early results were remarkably good, both from the point of view of pain relief as well as mobility. However, within the first 5 years, we observed signs of loosening of the humeral component in one third of all the operated cases. The removal of the loose prosthesis was not difficult to achieve, and the sine–sine arthroplasty which resulted thereafter showed a satisfactory stability and mobility due to the fact the humeral condyles and the ligaments had been preserved. This was at least a consolation, but not a justification to continue with this type of prosthesis.

We carefully analyzed the stresses on the elbow prosthesis which might have caused the early loosening and found the following forces to be responsible for this type of failure (Fig. 2):

1. Vertical stresses which favor the subsidence of the prosthesis between the humeral condyles when the patient leans on the extended arm.

2. Forces of rotation becoming important mainly during pronation and supination and even more so when using the arm in an abducted position, where the long lever of the forearm reaches a value 100 times greater than the intramedullary fixation.
3. Perhaps the most important stress arises when lifting a weight with flexed elbow. The resultant force runs nearly parallel to the ulna, which explains why loosening of the ulnar component only occurs exceptionally, whereas the stresses on the dorsal humeral wall typically cause a migration of the humeral prosthesis in a dorsal direction, with perforation of the wall and migration of the end of the stem in an opposite, ventral direction.

The conclusion drawn from this study motivated our team to construct a new prosthesis which maintained the minimal bone resection between the condyles,

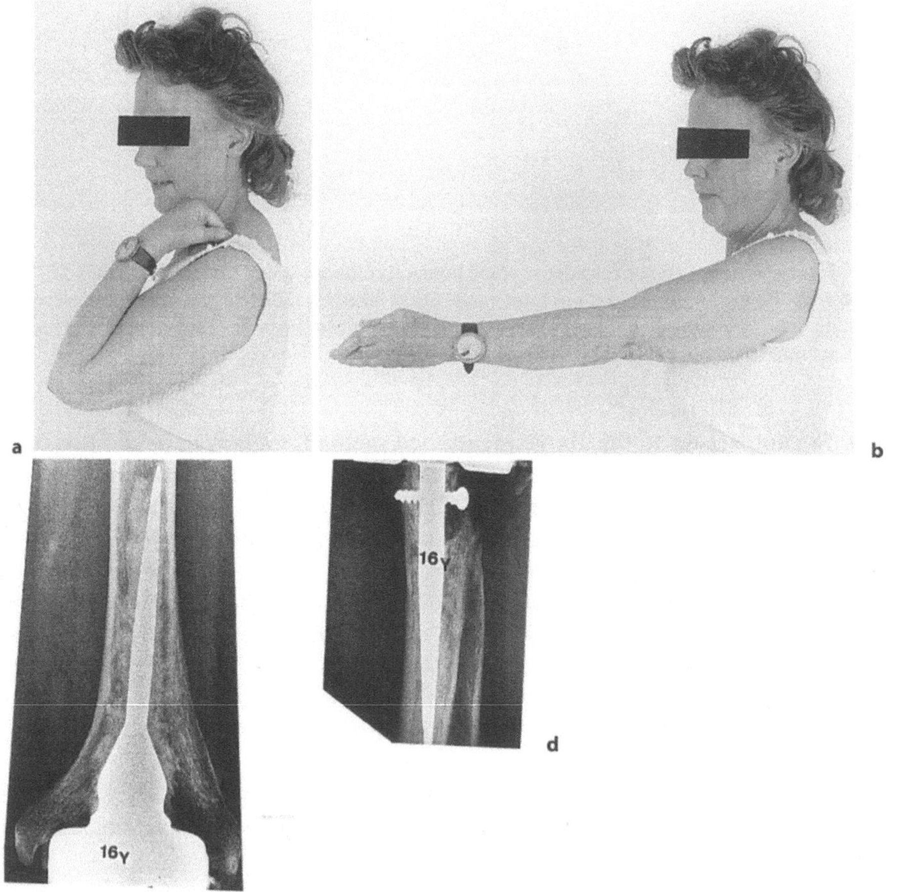

Fig. 3. Sixteen years after implantation of a GSB II elbow prosthesis, there is no sign of aseptic loosening in spite of still excellent mobility and full use of the elbow

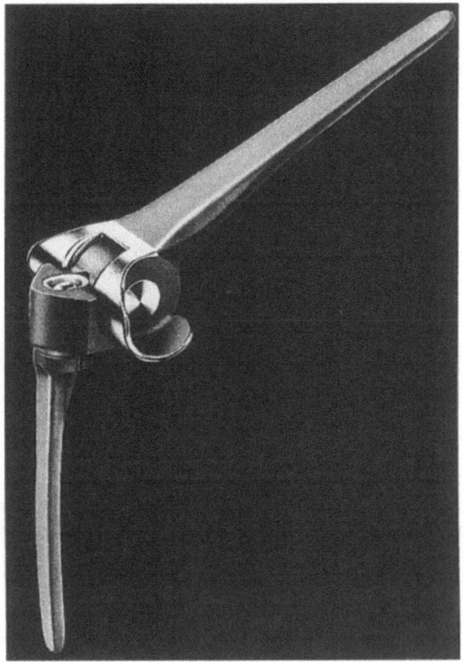

Fig. 4. GSB III prosthesis, a sloppy hinge with flanges on the distal and anterior part, resting on the humeral condyles. There is a clearance between the humeral and ulnar component of about 4°

but added flanges to the prosthesis resting on the anterior part of the humeral condyles, thereby compensating the force mentioned in item 3 above. Another flange resting on the distal surface of the humeral condyle acts against all stresses which may cause subsidence. With this new principle of construction, the GSB II prosthesis was still a rigid metal-to-metal hinge joint and was used in only two patients, one of whom has since died. The second patient, 16 years after surgery, still enjoys full activity of the elbow, which shows no signs of loosening. In 1978 we added to the principle of the GSB II prosthesis (Fig. 3) a slow friction principle (Fig. 4) by covering the axle with polyethylene bushes. The part which assembles both components also has a metal-to-polyethylene contact as well as a clearance of 4°. This sloppy hinge allows the ligamentous and muscular structures to reduce the stresses upon the interface.

Operative Technique

The operative technique is of particular importance for the success of any type of artificial elbow joint. Our own technique differs from others right from the beginning in the choice of operative approach. We use a transtricipital approach (Fig. 5) [4] in which the extensor mechanism is split proximal to the olecranon and detached in a longitudinal direction with thin bone slivers from the olecranon and the posterior 3–4 cm of the dorsal wall of the ulna by means of a sharp

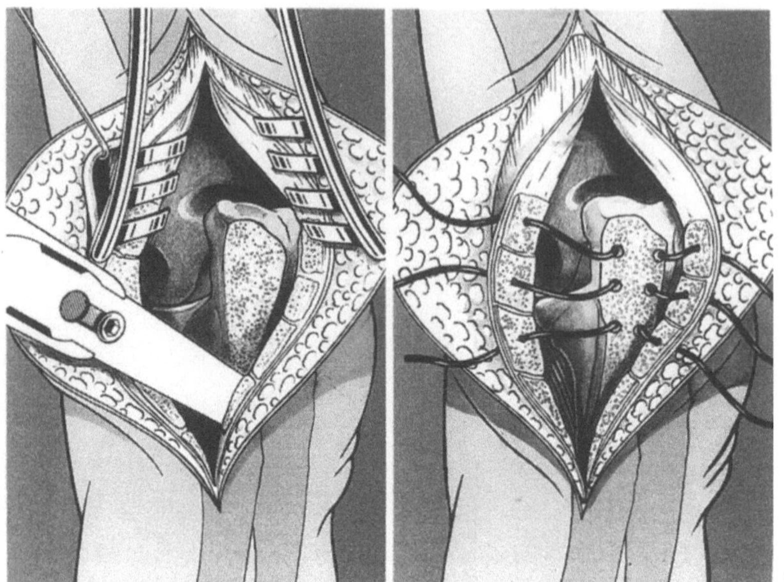

Fig. 5a,b. Our transtricipital approach to the elbow which detaches the tendon from the olecranon with thin bone slivers, preserving the continuity of the extensor mechanism

Ombredanne (Synthes, Bettlach, Switzerland) chisel. This enables us to maintain a solid continuity of the extensor mechanism and to refix the extensor apparatus safely to the ulna. Moreover, this approach allows an excellent view of the whole joint, avoids many possible complications, and is responsible for a minimal lack of active extension. The ulnar nerve is identified and mobilized down to the first muscular branch, protecting its vascular supply. We consider resection of the sharp edge of the anterior and ulnar articular surface (where normally the anterior ulnar collateral ligament is inserted) to be of particular importance, as it lies in the immediate vicinity of the ulnar nerve. In many cases, if it has not been resected right from the beginning of the operation, we suspect that this bone spicule is one of the causes of ulnar nerve lesions during manipulation of the arm, lesions which have been reported in the literature to be particularly frequent. This risk is even greater when the nerve has not been identified and mobilized. Sacrificing the anterior fibers of the ulnar collateral ligament is of no importance in our GSB III prosthesis, as the prosthesis has inbuilt stability.

Results

When discussing results with elbow arthroplasty, it is necessary to clarify whether we are presenting an analysis of cases suffering from rheumatoid arthritis (RA; the great majority in most statistics in the literature) or whether we are dealing with

Table 1. GSB III elbow arthroplasty in rheumatoid arthritis patients from 1978 to 1992 ($n = 118$): patients' characteristics

Side (%)	
Right	48
Left	24
Bilateral	28
Sex (%)	
Female	81
Male	19
Mean age at operation	56.8
(years)	
Follow-up (years)	
Maximum	14.0
Mean	4.3

Table 2. Preoperative X-ray findings

	Joints (%)
Larsen stage 5	64
Larsen stage 4	30
Ankylosis	4
Sine-sine	1
Fracture	1

cases of post-traumatic osteoarthritis (OA) in which previous operations to stabilize compound fractures have already been performed before arthroplasty. These previous operations and the extensive scarring (due to the trauma and the previous operation) as well as deformities and anatomic distortion make the operative procedure particularly difficult and are therefore responsible for an increased complication rate. Accordingly, we do not expect the same range of motion as in RA cases. We therefore intend to present the results with RA patients and OA patients separately.

From 1978 to the end of 1993, we implanted 187 GSB III elbow joints, 152 in RA patients and 35 in patients suffering from post-traumatic OA. The analysis presented in this article concerns 144 operations performed between 1978 and March 1992; 118 were RA patients and 81% were women (Table 1). In the post-traumatic OA group, there was an equal distribution of female and male patients. The main indication for operation was pain. The X-rays showed well-advanced destruction, corresponding in two thirds of all the cases to Larsen-Dahle-Eek stage 5 (Table 2). In 26% of cases, previous surgery had been performed.

Pain relief (Fig. 6) was obtained in the great majority of cases in both groups. The range of motion improved in both groups (Table 3), the gain being even more considerable in the post-traumatic cases, considering the worse preoperative situation. The extensor deficit is insignificant, particularly in the RA cases, compared

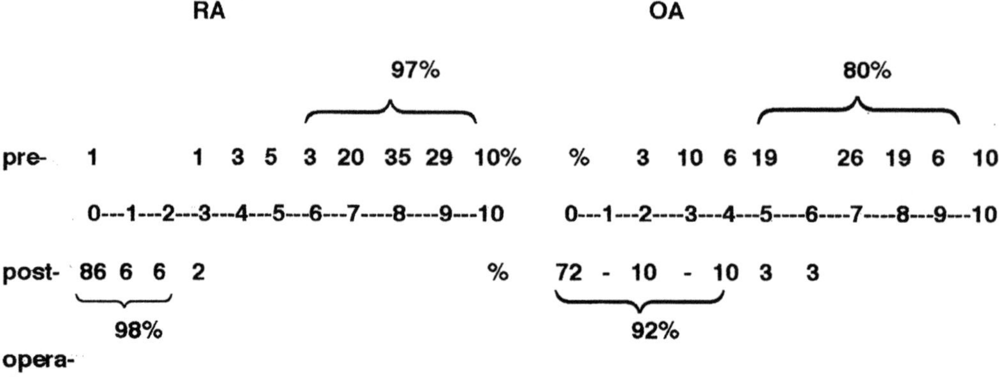

Fig. 6. Pain scale (0, no pain; 10, very severe pain). *RA*, rheumatoid arthritis; *OA*, osteoarthritis

Table 3. Comparison of range of motion before and after the operation

	Rheumatoid arthritis patients			Osteoarthritis patients		
	Preoperative	Postoperative	Gain	Preoperative	Postoperative	Gain
Flexion	118°	134°	28°	95°	126°	37°
Extension	−38°	−26°		−40°	−34°	
Pronation	54°	67°	25°	55°	73°	36°
Supination	50°	62°		49°	67°	

to most statistics in the literature. This may be due mainly to our operative approach (see above). The range of motion depends (especially in the post-traumatic OA cases) largely on the preoperative clinical and radiologic situation; it is reduced in all those cases where previous operations (osteosynthesis, several attempts to heal the fractures, etc.) have produced extensive scarring or, as in the case shown in Fig. 7, pseudarthrosis with shortening of the bones and extensive retraction of the soft tissues was present. Accordingly, even severe post-traumatic cases without previous surgery have a better result (Fig. 8).

Complications

The percentage of complications with elbow arthroplasty published in the international literature [5–23] is extraordinarily high: 357 out of 828 cases, i.e., 43% of all published cases. Late complications occurred in 23% of cases. Analysis of our own cases reveals a much lower percentage in the RA cases (Table 4). In the post-traumatic OA cases, the rate of complication is significantly higher. The complications occurring most frequently include loosening, ulnar nerve lesions,

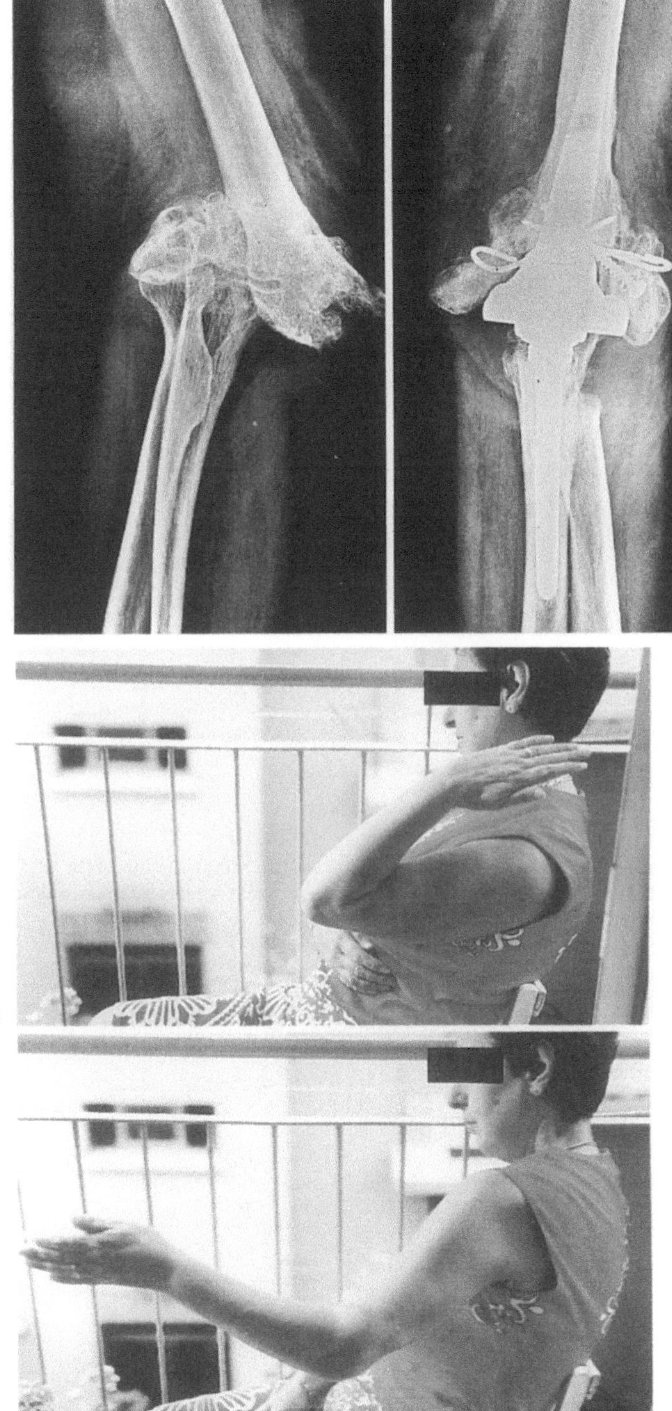

Fig. 7a,b. Post-traumatic osteoarthritis with pseudarthrosis after several previous unsuccessful operations. The reconstruction of the humeral condyles and implantation of the GSB III prosthesis led to solid bone healing. **c,d** In this patient there is extensive scar formation and we cannot expect a better extension; the triceps, having been damaged, does not glide normally on the posterior wall of the humerus and cannot transmit its full power to the olecranon. The patient is happy with the useful flexion and also because she suffers no more pain

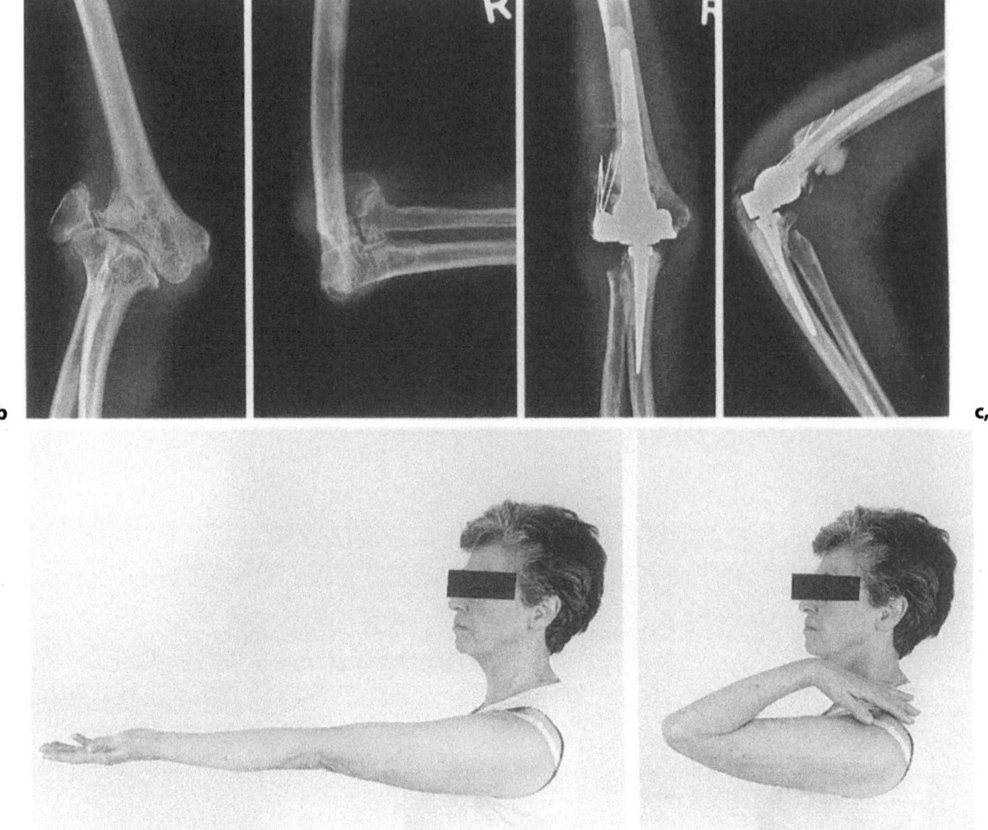

Fig. 8a,b. This post-traumatic patient had no previous surgery. **c,d** After implantation of the GSB III prosthesis and reconstruction of the humeral condyle. **e,f** Excellent result 4 years after operation in spite of difficult preoperative conditions

Table 4. Complications at our clinic

Complication	No. of joints
Ulnar nerve lesion	1
Fracture ulnar epicondyle	2
Disassembly	5[a]
Infections	3[b]
Spontaneously healing blisters	2
Total	13

Complications occurred in 13 out of 118 rheumatoid arthritis patients (11%) and nine out of 26 osteoarthritis patients.

[a] Fractured olecranon, $n = 2$.

[b] Superficial, $n = 1$.

Table 5. Aseptic loosening reported in the literature (1986–1992)

Type	Elbow joints (%)
Radiologic	17.2
Humerus	12.1
Ulna	5.1
Clinical	6.4
Humerus	3.7
Ulna	2.7

infections, and dislocations or disassembling of the two components of the prosthesis.

Loosening

The frequency of radiologic and clinical loosening which we found in the literature (1986–1992) is shown in Table 5. The number of aseptic loosenings of the GSB III prosthesis is extremely low. It occurred in four out of 118 (3.3%) cases in the RA group and in two out of 26 (7.6%) cases in the post-traumatic OA group. So far we have had to revise the prosthesis in only two post-traumatic patients for aseptic loosening. One of these patients (shown in Fig. 9) is of particular interest: three operations had been performed for intra-articular condylar fracture and pseudarthrosis before we implanted the GSB III prosthesis. Thereafter, the patient performed heavy manual labor and, after a few years, developed an aseptic loosening with extraordinary thinning of the cortical bone and spontaneous fracture. We replaced the loose humeral component using a new humeral component with a conic stem with conic flanges according to the Wagner hip revision prosthesis. This humeral component was implanted without cement. We were astonished to see how fast new bone developed spontaneously with no further sign of component loosening.

Of particular interest is our survey of 47 elbows in 43 patients who underwent operations 10–16 years ago; 14 patients (15 elbows operated on) have since died and two patients (from Yugoslavia and Sicily) were lost to follow-up. All other patients were examined personally, clinically, and with X-rays. In only three patients were signs of progressive radiolucency due to an aseptic loosening found (Fig. 10).

Ulnar Nerve Lesions

In the international literature from 1986 to 1992, ulnar nerve lesions were found in 10.8% of the cases. We had only 2% in our own series and only in one case was it necessary to perform a nerve suture. We feel that the use of our approach and the

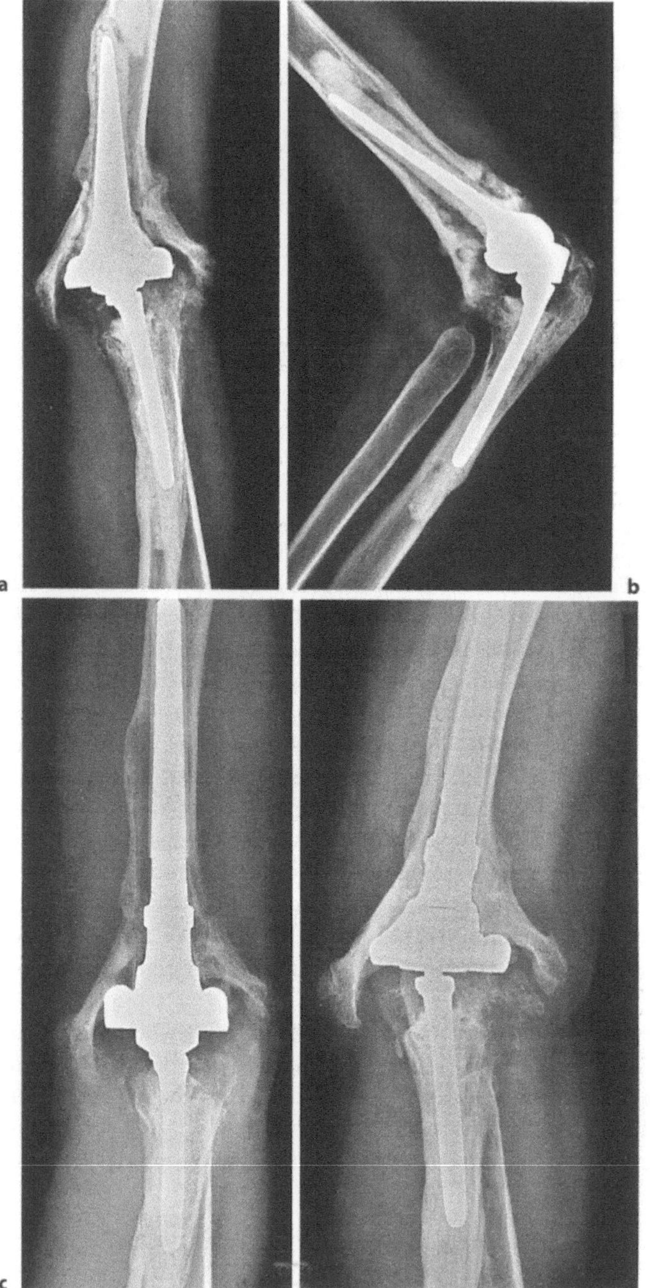

Fig. 9a,b. Post-traumatic osteoarthritis in a manual worker. Loosening of the GSB III prosthesis a few years after implantation. **c** Revision with a special GSB III prosthesis; noncemented concial titanium stem with conical fins. **d** Bone has spontaneously become thicker. Solid fixation of the prosthesis

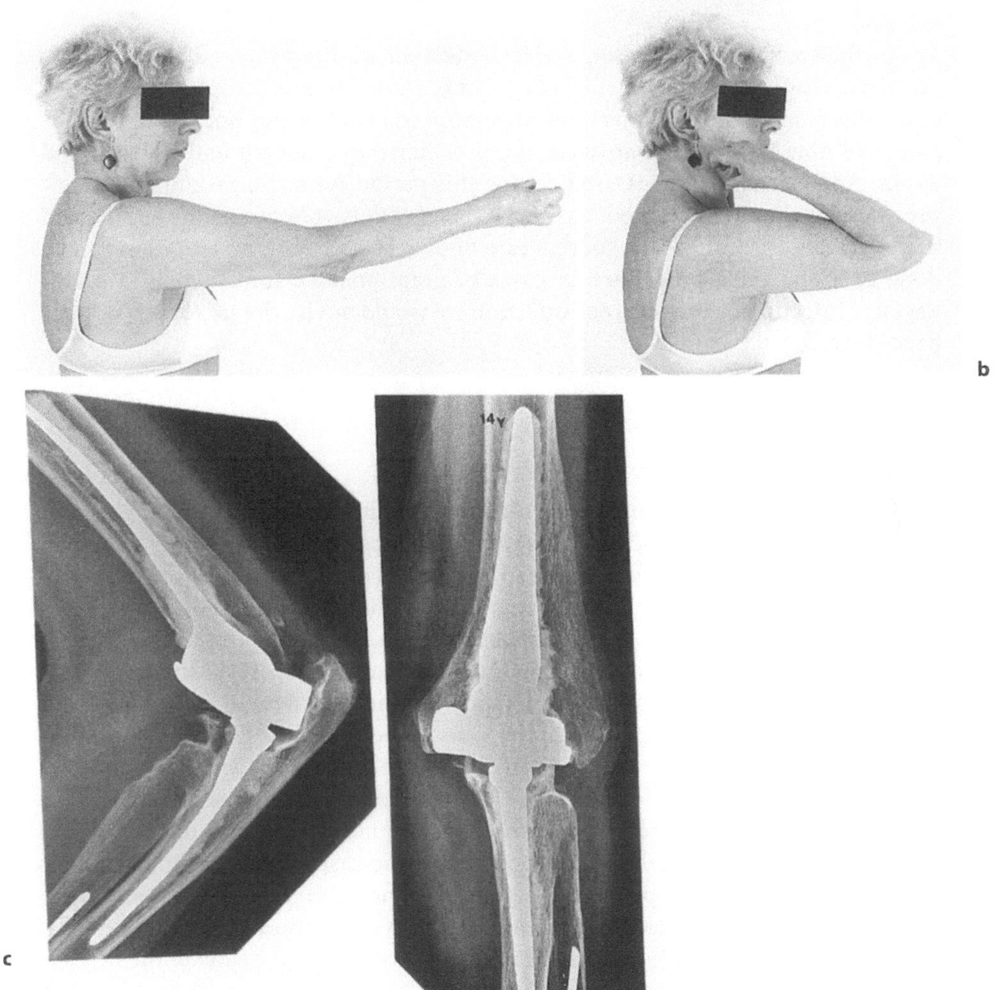

Fig. 10a,b. Fourteen years after implantation of bilateral GSB III elbows in a rheumatoid arthritis patient. The clinical picture shows excellent and painless function on both sides. **c,d** The X-ray shows no radiologic loosening

mobilization of the ulnar nerve and resection of the sharp ulnar edge on the articular surface of the ulna are the main reasons for the low incidence of ulnar nerve problems.

Infections

In the international literature from 1986 to 1992, infections were found in 8.1%, and 4.8% were deep infections. We had three infections in our cases of RA patients (corresponding to 2.5%) and only one in the post-traumatic cases (corresponding to 3.8%).

In the early years, in cases of deep infection we used to remove the elbow prosthesis and convert the arthroplasty into a sine–sine arthroplasty. In a few cases, this resulted in an elbow joint with reduced stability, but not too significant pain. We now favor the removal of the prosthesis and cement and wait for 6–8 weeks. An external fixator is used during this period for stabilization, and a new prosthesis is then reimplanted. Our experience with such a procedure in infected knee prostheses resulted in a success rate of over 80%. The reimplantation can be done as a one-stage procedure in cases of gram-positive infection. In a gram-negative infection or in recurrent infection we would advise the use of a two-stage procedure.

Instability

In the international literature from 1986 to 1992, instability was found in 7.1%; 4.3% were dislocations, 2.2% subluxations. This complication is only found in nonlinked prostheses and is associated with excessively extensive soft tissue release or with neglect of the carrying angle. Sloppy hinges have a inherent stability and may therefore only show an uncoupling or disassembling of the two components. This phenomenon is found in the literature in 5%–10%. In most cases polyethylene wear of the snap-fit mechanism was the reason for uncoupling. In our GSB III prosthesis, disassembling of the two components was the main complication in the RA and post-traumatic cases. We found it in 4% in the RA patients and 15.3% in the post-traumatic cases. Excessively extensive soft tissue release and the fact that the rotation center of the prosthesis did not correspond to the original center were the main causes. In the post-traumatic cases it may be impossible to define the rotation center properly; therefore, an increased rate of disassembling is to be expected in comparison to the RA patients. We now use a device to treat these cases in a relatively simple manner or in high-risk cases, at the time of the original arthroplasty, to prevent disassembling; the device lengthens the connecting piece of the ulnar component, therefore preventing this component slipping out of the humeral component.

Revisions

The number of revisions with any prosthesis reflects the long-term success rate of the presented method. The revision rate was 18% in the international literature (1986–1992) and the rate of permanent complications was 15%, in spite of revision. Our own revision rate amounted to only 8.4%. The permanent complication rate was 3.4% in the RA group and significantly higher (15.3%) in the post-traumatic cases. Tables 6 and 7 show the reasons for revision and the type of lasting compli-

Table 6. Reasons for revisions

Complication	Type of revision	Joints (n)
RA patients		
Disassembly	–	4
Fractured ulnar epicondyle	Osteosynthesis	3
Perforation of ulna	Sine-sine arthroplasty	1
Infection	Sine-sine arthroplasty	2
Total	–	10 (8.4%)
OA patients		
Disassembly	Sine-sine arthroplasty ($n = 2$), proximalization of ulnar component ($n = 2$)	4
Ectopic bone formation	Removal	2
Loosening	New GSB III prosthesis	1
Stem perforation	New GSB III prosthesis	1
Total	–	8 (30.7%)

RA, rheumatoid arthritis; OA, osteoarthritis.

Table 7. Lasting complications

Complication	Joints (n)
RA patients	
None	9
Residual ulnar nerve symptoms	2
Sine-sine arthroplasty	2
Total	13 (3.4%)
OA patients	
None	5
Sine-sine arthroplasty	2
Ulnar nerve irritation	1
Carpal tunnel syndrome	1
Total	9 (15.3)

RA, rheumatoid arthritis; OA, osteoarthritis.

cations. We must add that, with the exception of two patients, all those in whom we had to remove the GSB III prosthesis and convert the elbow into a sine–sine arthroplasty considered the result to be satisfactory and felt that the situation was still better than it was preoperatively.

Conclusion

In conclusion, careful analysis of a closed series of patients receiving the GSB III prosthesis, of which the earliest cases were operated on 16 years ago, shows that good or excellent results were achieved in 93%. In 92% of cases, patients were satisfied and said that they would repeat the operation again under the same circumstances. We therefore feel that the long-term results are already comparable to those obtained with knee and hip arthroplasty.

References

1. Ollier LX (1978) De la résection du coude dans les cas d'ankylose. Rev Med Chir 6:12
2. Hass J (1930) Die Mobilisierung ankylotischer Ellbogen- und Kniegelenke mittels Arthroplastik. Langenbecks Arch Klin Chir 160:693
3. Gschwend N (1977) Die operative Behandlung der chronischen Polyarthritis. Thieme, Stuttgart, p 55
4. Gschwend N (1981) Our operative approach to the elbow joint. Arch Orthop Traum Surg 98:143–146
5. Brumfield RH, Volz RG, Green JF (1981) Total elbow arthroplasty, a clinical review of 30 cases employing the Mayo and AHSC prostheses. Clin Orthop 158:137–141
6. Dennis DA, Clayton ML, Ferlic DC, Stringer EA, Bramlett KW (1990) Capitello-condylar total elbow arthroplasty for rheumatoid arthritis. J Arthroplasty 5[Suppl]:S83–S88
7. Figgie HE, Inglis AE, Mow C (1986) Total Elbow Arthroplasty in the face of significant bone stock or soft tissue losses. Proc R Soc Med 62:1031–1035
8. Figgie MP, Inglis AE, Mow CS, Figgie HE III (1989) Total elbow arthroplasty for complete ankylosis of the elbow. J Bone Joint Surg [Am] 71:513–520
9. Friedman RJ, Ewald FC (1987) Arthroplasty of the ipsilateral shoulder and elbow in patients who have rheumatoid arthritis. J Bone Joint Surg [Am] 69:661–667
10. Goldberg VM, Figgie HE III, Inglis AE, Figgie MP (1988) Current concepts review, total elbow arthroplasty. J Bone Joint Surg [Am] 70:778–783
11. Gschwend N (1991) The case for a linked elbow prosthesis. In: Hämäläinen MJ, Hagena FW (eds) Rheumatoid arthritis surgery of the elbow. Karger, Basel, pp 98–112 (Rheumatology, vol 15)
12. Jonsson B, Larsson SE (1990) Elbow arthroplasty in rheumatoid arthritis. Function after 1–2 years in 20 cases. Acta Orthop Scand 61:344–347
13. Kudo H (1985) Long term follow-up study of total elbow arthroplasty with nonconstrained prosthesis. In: Kashiwagi D (ed) Elbow joint, proceedings of the international seminar Kobe, Japan, congress series 678. Excerpta Medica International, Amsterdam, pp 269–276
14. Morrey BF, Bryan RS (1987) Revision total elbow arthroplasty. J Bone Joint Surg [Am] 69:523–532
15. Roper BA, Tuke M, O'Riordan SM, Bulstrode CJ (1986) A new unconstrained elbow. A prospective review of 60 replacements. J Bone Joint Surg [Br] 68:566–569
16. Rozing PM, Poll RG (1991) Use of the Souter-Strathclyde total elbow prosthesis in patients who have rheumatoid arthritis. J Bone Joint Surg [Am] 73:1227–1233
17. Sourmelis SG, Burke FD, Varian JPW (1986) A review of total elbow arthroplasty and an early assessment of the Liverpool elbow prosthesis. J Hand Surg 11-B:407–413
18. Swanson AB, De Groot-Swanson G, Masada K, Makino M, Pires PR, Gannon DM, Sattel AB (1991) Constrained total elbow arthroplasty. J Arthroplasty 6:203–212
19. Trancik T, Wilde AH, Borden LS (1987) Capitellocondylar total elbow arthroplasty. Clin Orthop Related Res 223:175–180
20. TrepmanE, Ewald FC (1991) Early failure of silicone radial head implants in the rheumaoid elbow. A complication of silicone radial head implant arthroplasty. J Arthroplasty 6:59–65
21. Weiland AJ, Weiss APC, Willis RP, Moore JR (1989) Capitellocondylar total elbow replacement. A long-term follow-up study. J Bone Joint Surg [Am] 71:217–222
22. Wilde AH (1992) Captillocondylar total elbow replacement. A long-term follow-up study. J Bone Joint Surg [Am] 74:95–100
23. WolfeSW, Ranawat CS (1990) The osteo-anconeus flap. J Bone Joint Surg [Am] 72:684–688

Elbow Replacement Arthroplasty for Flail and Ankylosed Elbows

A.E. Inglis

Introduction

This paper will concern itself with the two extremes of elbow problems. First, I will review the results for stiff and ankylosed elbows and second, with flail or unstable elbows. Each of these represent unusual and challenging anatomic problems [4]. The ankylosed elbow partly represents an excess of anatomic resources, whereas the flail or unstable elbow represents a paucity or damaged anatomical resources. In both situations, there are serious functional and disabling problems which must be addressed by the surgeon [3].

Stiff and Ankylosed Elbows

Studies of total elbow replacement for elbow problems including stiff elbows have been reported in the literature [9–12]. However, the first publication which discussed total replacement arthroplasty for a complete ankylosis as a single diagnosis did not appear until 1989 [6]. The authors presented a series of 16 patients in which 19 arthroplasties had been performed (in three patients the operation was bilateral). There were ten men (12 elbows) and six women (seven elbows). The average age was 34 years, with a range of 16–72 years. All of the elbows were completely ankylosed in flexion or extension. There were six elbows that still maintained pronation and supination. The duration of the ankylosis was an average of 5 years, ranging from 6 months to 16 years. Eight patients had juvenile rheumatoid arthritis, one patient had rheumatoid arthritis, two patients had ankylosing spondylitis, five patients had post-traumatic arthritis, and three patients had post-immobilization ankylosis.

A major indication for surgical therapy was bilateral ankylosis in which neither hand could be brought to the face or to the hips. An additional indication occurred where there was limited function in the opposite extremity and additional painless elbow flexion and extension was needed. The final indication was an isolated ankylosis which severely limited the use of the hand for the activities of daily living or a vocational activity that required the use of the hand. A contraindication was given in a patient who would predictably abuse the implant arthroplasty, e.g., repeated impact loading, or would have unrealistic expectations

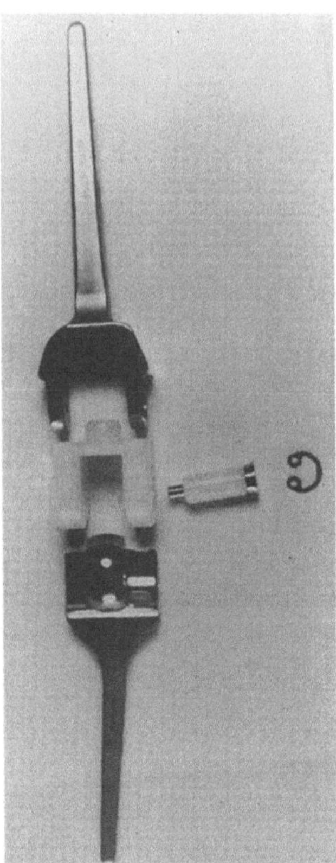

Fig. 1. Hospital for Special Surgery implant design manufactured by the Osteonics Corporation. It is centrally loaded with some loading on the two "condyles" at the extreme of varus and valgus. The axle is not loaded except at the extremes of tensile forces

of the surgical outcome, e.g., playing tennis. The average follow-up for this group of patients was almost 6 years, with a range of 2–12 years. No patients were lost to follow-up. Four types of implants were used in these arthroplasties. All of these four implants were of the Hospital for Special Surgery design with similar geometric and anatomic characteristics. All were linked and semiconstrained prostheses with 7° valgus and 7° varus laxity. The first was the Pritchard-Walker and was used in 1974 and 1975. The second was the snap-fit triaxial elbow replacement used between 1975 and 1980. The third was the Hospital for Special Surgery (Fig. 1) prosthesis. The final implant type was custom implants. These were fabricated both at The Hospital for Special Surgery and by the Osteonics company (Allendale, NJ, USA).

Surgical Technique

Initially, the Campbell triceps-detaching technique was used [2]. In 1980 this was replaced by the Bryan Morrey surgical approach [1]. A sterile tourniquet was used uniformly throughout the procedure. The use of a sterile tourniquet permits a more generous proximal incision, particularly in short upper arms. It also allows an access to the tourniquet if there are any technical problems, such as the need to extend the incision more proximally. This incision is a posteromedial approach with the combined structures of the triceps muscle and the epimysium of the ulnar flexor muscle of the wrist, the periosteum of the ulna, the epimysium of the anconeus, and the radial extensor muscle of the wrist all being reflected laterally as a single layer. The ulnar nerve is retracted carefully with a rubber Penrose drain. The radial head is uniformly resected to insure that there is no radial head interference with the remaining capitellum. Any additional irregularities in the remaining radius must be removed to assure that there is no interference in the proximal radioulnar joint that would restrict pronation and supination. The arm is carefully rotated to assure that there are no remaining osteophytes or sharp edges to impinge on the ulnar side of the proximal radioulnar joint. The resection of the radial head is always proximal to the annular ligament.

At this point in the surgical approach, it is necessary to carefully define the ankylosed ulnohumeral joint. Therefore, the periosteum and the muscle attachments adjacent to the ulnohumeral joint are carefully elevated. When these structures are elevated it is relatively easy to define the entire joint line even in the ankylosed joint. The entire joint is then opened either with narrow osteotomes driven in only 3 or 4 mm or through the cortex; a microsagittal saw with a narrow blade or small burrs can also be used to open up the margins of the joint. This must be done circumferentially around the entire ulnohumeral joint. Once this cortical surface has been opened, it is safe to gently manipulate the elbow into flexion. There will be a distinct, but faint "crack" as the ulnohumeral joint is opened. Because the surrounding muscle origins and capsular remnants have been previously elevated and released, the ulna and humerus are easily separated for completion of the arthroplasty.

The center of rotation of the semilunar notch of the ulna is easily determined by placing a finger in the semilunar notch of the ulna and then marking the center of rotation of the joint. The appropriate amount of semilunar notch and coronoid process are marked with the ulnar template and then excised with microsagittal saws. A burr is then used to identify the intramedullary metaphyseal portion of the proximal ulnar metaphysis. The remaining medullary portion is then reamed and broached sufficiently so that the trial prosthesis can be inserted. The center of rotation of the trial ulnar-bearing system must be in line with the previously marked center of rotation of the semilunar notch of the ulna.

The humeral component is similarly prepared for the implant by marking the humerus using the humeral templates. The trochlea is then excised. The epicondylar bone is preserved, as only a minimal amount of metaphyseal bone including the edges of the coronoid and olecranon are excised to accommodate the hinge portion of the humeral prosthesis. The intramedullary cavity of the humerus is then gently reamed and broached sufficiently so that the humeral component can be inserted. The center of rotation of the humeral component again must be in line with the center of rotation of the distal humerus. The epicondyles are carefully preserved. Before cementing, trial implants are inserted into the ulna and humerus complete with the plastic bearing and the joint brought through a complete range of motion. The elbow should extend and flex fully without impingement. If there is insufficient extension, then more of the anterior capsule and/or a small amount of the bracheal muscle must be incised or more of the ulna or humerus must be resected until full extension can be achieved. Occasionally, a small amount of excessive epicondylar bone will remain distal to the humeral component; this is removed so that impingement is avoided. The cement is then prepared in a soft liquid form to facilitate packing into the ulna and humerus. Small amounts of methylene blue and tobramycin antibiotic are added to the cement. Both ulna and humerus are filled with cement at the same time. The components are then inserted into place, with the center of rotation of each of the components maintained as planned.

After the humeral and ulnar components have been cemented into place, a small hole is made in the lateral epicondyle with the special axle drill so that the axle can be inserted. The drill is held in line with a humeral drill guide. The ultrahigh molecular weight polyethylene bearing is then inserted over the top of the humeral component. The ulnar and humeral components are then articulated. The small metal axle and the high molecular weight polyethylene sleeve are put into position. The small metal axle is in the proper final position and is secure when a distinct locking "click" occurs. The tourniquet is released and hemostasis is secured before the triceps muscle is reattached. The tourniquet is then reinflated. Any remaining olecranon is removed if it protrudes beyond the ulnar component. The thickened central portion of the triceps tendon is sutured to the tip of the olecranon process with nonabsorbable sutures. The epimysium of the ulnar flexor muscle of the wrist is closed, The ulnar nerve is not transposed. A negative pressure drain is inserted and always sutured to the skin to prevent accidental removal during the final suturing and dressing procedures. Negative pressure drain is left in position for 24 h or until inactive. The patient is placed in a soft bulky compression dressing stabilized with an anterior splint at 45° of extension.

All dressings and splints are removed on the fourth postoperative day, and active flexion/extension and pronation/supination exercises are initiated. The occupational service rehabilitation protocol emphasizes the importance of active elbow flexion and passive elbow extension. Pronation and supination are similarly begun. At this point in time the elbow is placed in a removable posterior splint to hold the elbow either in flexion or extension at night or when not doing exercises (Fig. 2). The splint can easily be adjusted for a flexion or extension position with Velcro straps or removed for active exercise program.

Results

The patients were evaluated radiographically for stress shielding, heterotopic bone formation, implant migration, or loosening. The overall results were assessed using the Hospital for Special Surgery (HSS) scoring system [8]. This system

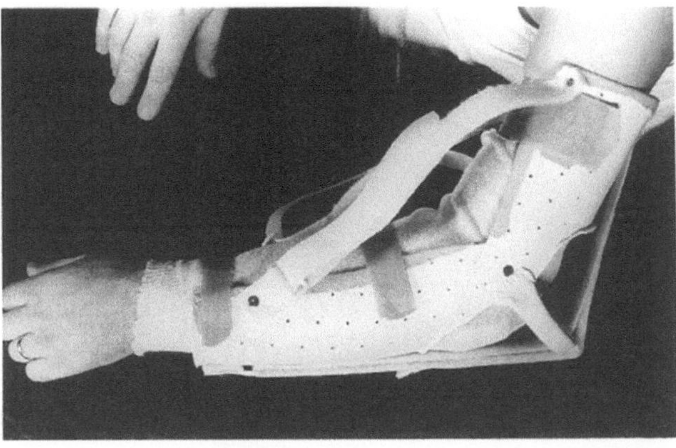

Fig. 2. Postoperative splint. Note the two Velcro straps in front of the splint and behind. They may be used alternatively to maintain the elbow post-operatively in flexion or extension. The splint is easily removed for exercises and therapy

strongly weights three areas, i.e., pain relief, function in terms of activities of daily living, and achieved arc of motion. Preoperatively, all patients were ankylosed and therefore had no flexion/extension arc. Postoperatively, they achieved an average arc of motion of 80° with a range of 30° 115°. The six patients with ankylosis of the ulnohumeral joint retained a preoperative arc of pronation and supination of 22° and postoperatively achieved an arc of pronation/supination of 90°. There were no radiolucent lines, no stress shielding, and no loosening or migration of any of the implants. Three elbows showed a grade I heterotopic bone formation. Using the HSS scoring system [8], 15 of 19 patients were rated good to excellent, and three patients were rated fair due to residual triceps muscle weakness. One patient was rated poor due to a deep infection.

During the period from 1974 to 1981, the Campbell triceps-detaching surgical approach was used in eight elbows [2]. In this group four would problems occurred and four patients required a postoperative manipulation. Eleven elbows were operated on in the period following 1981, during which time the Bryan Morrey approach was used. In this group there were no wound problems and none required manipulation. There was also an increase in the arc of motion.

Complications

There were three superficial infections that cleared without further surgical intervention. There was one deep infection. There was one asymptomatic fracture of an overhanging olecranon process (Fig. 3) and one ulnar nerve paresthesia that cleared quickly.

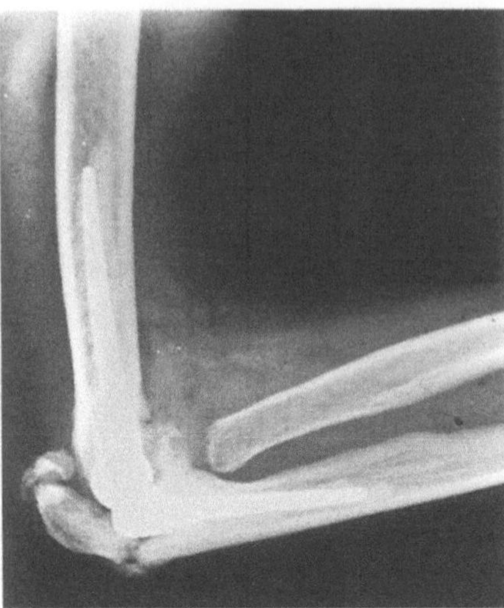

Fig. 3. Avulsion fracture of the olecranon process found at long-term follow-up. It was not asymptomatic and did not interfere with extension. We did not excise any redundant olecranon

Discussion

Ankylosis of the elbow is a severe disability, particularly when it is bilateral [6, 11]. Preoperatively, the unilateral patients, although they were pain free, had serious limitations in function. These functional limitations were frequently affected their work. The concept of operating on a painless elbow even in poor position is problematic. However, when this elbow seriously restricts overall hand function, then arthroplasty is a viable alternative. The youngest patient in this series was 15 years of age and had bilateral elbow ankylosis. He was not able to dress himself or to see to his daily hygiene. Following his bilateral elbow arthroplasties, he went on to attend college, medical school, and ultimately to become a radiologist. He is currently under active treatment 19 years after his bilateral elbow replacement arthroplasties. There was no implant loosening and no deterioration of the 80% good to excellent results with time. The three patients with triceps weakness were pain free and achieved a average arc of motion of 90° and were grateful for the improved hand function. The long-term results in this series of patients followed for up to 16 years with an average of more than 5 years were salutary and the complications minor.

Flail or Unstable Elbows

The flail or unstable elbow represents a different and perhaps more difficult therapeutic problem. The flail elbow is defined as one in which there is no active control of flexion or extension and the forearm hangs down no matter what position the upper arm assumes (Fig. 4). The unstable elbow is defined as one in which there is 45° or more medial and lateral instability (Fig. 5). There is also longitudinal

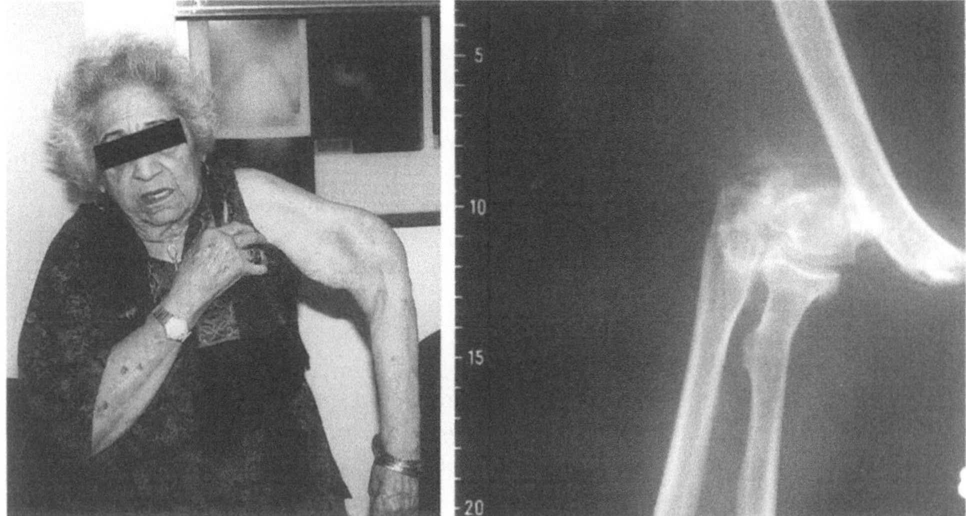

Fig. 4. a Patient with a flail elbow. She had a painful nonunited fracture with a normal shoulder and hand. The hand hung down in all positions of the upper arm. b Radiographs of the nonunited fracture

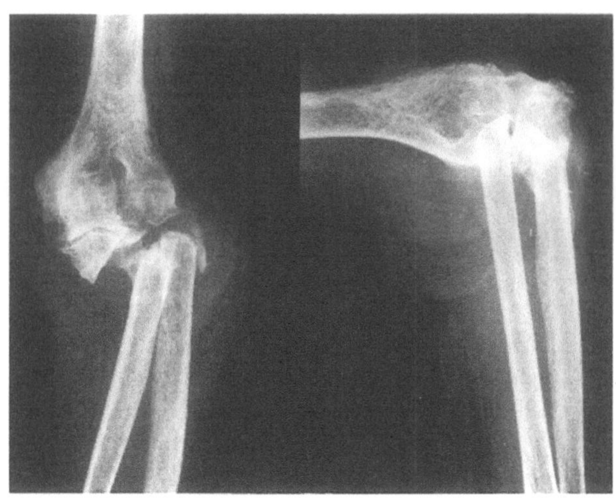

Fig. 5. Radiographs of an unstable elbow fracture in which there is a nonunion of an ulnar and radial fracture. There was gross medial and lateral instability. Patient also had an ankylosis of the ulnohumeral joint

instability or thromboning. Longitudinal instability also results in secondary loss of grasp power. This longitudinal weakness and instability occurs because as the elbow flexor and extensor muscles contract, they pull the forearm and hand proximally rather than into wrist and finger flexion and extension due to their epicondylar humeral origin.

Fundamentally, the loss of hand function is the major issue in these flail and unstable elbows, as it is a posit that the elbow postures the hand in space and positions the hand to or away from the body. Additionally, these patients even had pain at night, as the forearm would become tangled in the bed linen. As a rule, these patients with unstable and flail elbows will use the opposite hand to aid in posturing the affected hand. The obvious functional consequence is that the uninvolved hand is now involved in positioning the affected extremity instead of performing primary tasks of its own.

The therapeutic options for these patients are limited [5]. The surgeon may have another attempt at union, and indeed many patients in our series had multiple surgical attempts to attain bony union [13]. The surgeon may attempt an elbow arthrodesis for stabilization. Arthrodesis, however, is difficult to achieve [9, 12]. An elbow orthosis may be fabricated with hinges for medial and lateral stability [5, 7]. However, elbow arthrosis has not enjoyed high levels of patient compliance due to the difficulty of determining the center of normal rotation of the damaged joint and the fact that it is difficult to obtain a comfortable fit of the orthosis about the wrist and remaining malaligned epicondyles. Elbow replacement is sometimes the only remaining option.

The indications for surgery are uniformly pain and limitation of hand function. All patients in this series had been tried with braces, and multiple attempts had been made to achieve bony union. A contraindication to surgery is wound sepsis within 1 year. There were 21 patients in this series of flail and unstable elbows. Sixteen patients had nonunited fractures, three patients had rheumatoid arthritis with severe joint destruction, one patient had a traumatically absent elbow, and one patient had a neurologically absent elbow. The average age of these patients was 61 years, with a range of 31–79 years. Sixteen patients had prior operations, with an average of 2.3 operations per patient. One patient had six operations before the replacement arthroplasty. There were 21 patients (17 women and four men). The dominant hand was involved in 11 of 21 patients. All patients had normal or functional hands. There were four ulnohumeral ankyloses below a more proximal flail nonunion. These unstable pseudarthroses were in patients with long-standing supracondylar nonunions. Four implants were used in this study. The triaxial implant was used five times, the Hospital for Special Surgery implant was used four times and a custom implant was used 12 times. All of these implants had the same geometry or design characteristics, i.e., a long-stemmed humeral component with a 15° anterior angulation of the distal-bearing portion of the humeral implant. The ulnar component was fabricated with the normal 15° valgus angle. The bearing system was linked and semiconstrained and allowed 7° of valgus and 7° of varus laxity.

Meticulous preoperatve planning in concert with the implant manufacturers was required in those patients requiring a custom implant. Humeral shaft flutes were used to reduce rotation in certain patients. The use of flanges or sharp ridges about the humeral stem was helpful in those patients who were to have implants employing surfaces for bony ingrowth for fixation (Fig. 6). Additionally, implants were fabricated with holes in the distal humeral component for nonunited epicondylar attachment (Fig. 7). In patients with deficient metaphyseal bone or

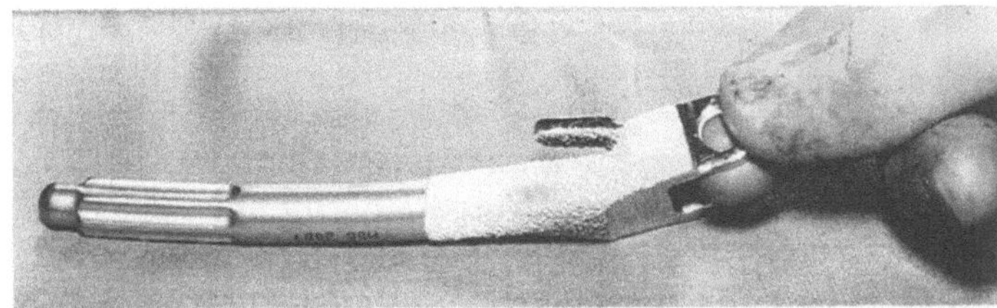

Fig. 6. Custom-made humeral component. Note the fluted stem for rotational stability. Porous coating has been added to the epicondylar area for biologic fixation. An anterior flange has been added for additional rotational stabilization. It was precisely fabricated to match the reamed humeral canal

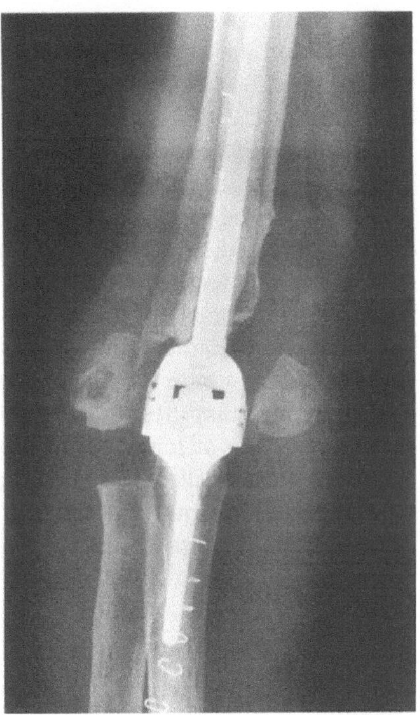

Fig. 7. Custom-made implant with holes in the distal portion of the humeral component for suture attachment of the epicondyles. The epicondylar fragments with their muscular attachments became securely attached and had not moved at long-term follow-up

when the humerus was merely a thin tube or the epicondylar flares were deficient, anterior flanges were added (Fig. 6). The remaining patients had preoperative planning with implant templates for study by X-ray.

Surgical Technique

The Campbell triceps release was used in surgery until 1981; thereafter the Bryan Morrey [1] approach was used. The soft tissue dissection and management was frequently difficult due to the presence of multiple previous incisions; however, the same concept of only one deep flap and meticulous soft tissue care was followed. The distal humeral fragment was carefully preserved in those cases of ulnohumeral ankylosis following supracondylar fractures of the humerus. The same technique of separating the ankylosed ulnohumeral joint was used as in the ulnohumeral ankylosis cases. However, after separating the ulnohumeral ankylosed segment the central trochlear portion of the humeral fragment was excised to make space for the distal portion of the humeral prosthetic component. In those cases where the proximal humeral fragment was tubular or the remaining epicondyles were small or absent, an anterior flange was added to the humeral component. The remaining two epicondyles with their muscular attachments were preserved and prepared to be sutured to the humeral component. Again, the ulnar nerve was not transposed. Rehabilitation was initiated on the fourth postoperative day or when the wound was dry, and the arm was splinted similarly to those patients undergoing surgery for ankylosed elbows.

Technical caveats were noted in this group of patients. Additional time was frequently required for isolation of the ulnar nerve, which was encased in dense scar tissue, callus, or bone. Additional time may be required to take down an ankylosis of the ulnohumeral joint. The epicondylar fragments should be preserved, trimmed, and prepared to be attached to the humeral component. These fragments are secured by sutures through the prepared holes (Fig. 7) in the humeral component or by a sling created by sutures around the back of the humeral component. Although these epicondylar fragments were not intended to achieve bony union to the nearby humerus, sufficient fibrous stabilization occurred such that these epicondylar fragments maintained their original postoperative position at long-term follow-up. Restoring the origins of the flexor and extensor muscles allows for their torsional protection of the cement–bone bond of the humeral implant. A full range of motion should be achieved before the components are finally cemented into place. Avoidance of hematoma should be a high-priority item with fully functional negative pressure drains that are sutured to the skin.

Results

In 81%, good to excellent results were found at long-term follow-up. The patients with bearing failure due to dissociation of the snap-fit triaxial prosthesis were reoperated upon and the failures were ultimately corrected with a new bearing and yoke, achieving excellent results. Two patients were rated as fair due to triceps muscle weakness. One patient developed loosening of a porous-coated humeral implant (Fig. 8). This was corrected with a long-stemmed cemented implant (Fig. 9). This patient was also rated as excellent at 2-year follow-up. One patient developed a deep infection following the replacement. She was operated upon 6 months following another replacement arthroplasty that had been removed for infection. She had a resection arthroplasty and is now in the same position as she was before her implant arthroplasty and is rated as a failure.

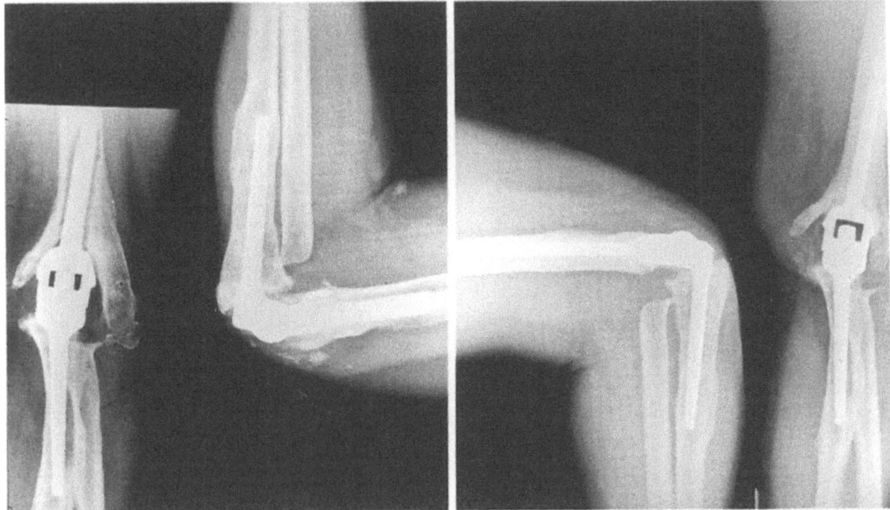

Fig. 8. Porous humeral and ulnar components in a young patient with a long-standing nonunion with old fractures in the ulna as well as the radius. The ulnar component achieved biologic fixation; however, the humeral component was too short and loosened

Fig. 9. This patient was revised to a long-stemmed cemented component and is asymptomatic

Complications

Five patients required reoperation. Four of these patients were restored to good to excellent status. Three of these patients had an early triaxial implant in which there was a bearing failure due to dissociation. These were corrected with a yoke that prevented further dissociation and ultimately achieved an excellent result. The one implant loosening occured in a patient with a custom-fabricated implant in which the porous-coated humeral stem was initially designed too short. This was corrected with a long-stemmed comented implant (Fig. 9). One patient developed a deep infection after a prior implant arthroplasty; only 6 months had elapsed between the two operations. She was revised to a resection arthroplasty and was rated as a failure.

Discussion

The flail or unstable elbow not only limits the function of the hand, but also limits the function of the opposite extremity, as it is frequently needed to position the affected elbow, thereby reducing it own effectiveness. The therapeutic options for patients with a flail or unstable elbow are limited. Arthrodesis would be a solution to instability; however, it is difficult to achieve, particularly in patients with such limited damage to anatomic resources [7, 9, 12, 13]. The results in this study suggest that, with careful planning, good to excellent results can be achieved in over 80% of cases.

Comment

Implant arthroplasty for both ankylosis and flail elbows is technically demanding; however, the complication rate was low at long-term follow-up and 85% of patients were able to reach their head and to carry out all activities of daily life. The relief of pain and stability were satisfactory in these patients. In both those patients with ankylosed and those with flail elbows, good, lasting functional results can be expected with total elbow replacement arthroplasty.

References

1. Bryan RS, Morrey BF (1982) Extensive posterior expposure of the elbow: a triceps-sparing approach. Clin Orthop 166:188
2. Campbell WC (1932) Incision for exposure of the elbow Joint. Am J Surg 15:65–67
3. Coonrad RW (1982) Seven year follow-up of coonrad total elbow replacemnt. In: Inglis AE (ed) Symposium on total joint replacement of the upper extremity. Mosby, St Louis
4. Ewald FC, Jacobs MA (1984) Total elbow arthoplasty. Clin Orthop 182:137–142
5. Figgie MD, Inglis AE, Mow CS, Figgie HE III (1989) Salvage of non-union of supracondylar fracture of the humerus by total elbow arthroplasty. J Bone Joint Surg 71 A:1058–1065
6. Figgie MP, Inglis AE, Mow CS, Figgie HE III (1989) Total elbow arthroplasty for ankylosis of the elbow. J Boen Joint Surg. 74(4):513–520
7. Inglis AE (1985) Rheumatoid arthritis. In: Morrey BF (ed) The elbow and its disorders Saunders; Philadelphia, pp 638–655
8. Inglis AE, Pellicci PM (1980) Total elbow replacement (J Bone Joint Surg) 62A:1252
9. Kock M, Lipscomb PR (1967) Arthrodesis of the elbow Clin Orthop 50:151
10. Kudo, Hiroshi, Ivano, Kunio (1990) Total elbow arthroplasty with a non-constrained surface replacement in patient who have rheumatoid arthritis, a long term follow-up study. J Bone Joint Surg 72A:355–365
11. Morrey BF (1988) Surgical takedown of the ankylosed elbow. Orthop. Trans. 12:734
12. Rashhoff, E, Burkhalter WE (1986) Arthrodesis of the salvaged elbow. Orthopedics 9(5):733
13. Schatzker J (1990) Intra-articular malnunions and non-unions (elbow). Orthop Clin North Am 21(4):743–757

Coonrad-Morrey Semiconstrained Total Elbow Arthroplasty

S.W. O'Driscoll and B.F. Morrey

Introduction

The Mayo-modified Coonrad total elbow prosthesis (Coonrad-Morrey) is a semiconstrained elbow replacement manufactured from Titanium Ti-6AI-4V alloy with a cobalt chrome pin that passes through the ultrahigh molecular weight polyethylene bushings to secure the ulnar component. This provides a "loose-hinge" mechanism. The metallic pin is secured with a split-locking ring. Uncoupling of this device during use has not occurred, and the prosthesis is easily disassembled if desired.

The theoretical advantage of this semiconstrained design has been confirmed by O'Driscoll and colleagues, who showed that the articulation tracks within the limits of its tolerance and it behaves as a true "semiconstrained" joint (Fig. 1). This decreases stresses on the bone-cement interface [14]. Markedly improved clinical results attest to the effectiveness of semiconstrained implants [2, 6, 8, 9, 12].

Of equal significance is the fact that the articulated implant dramatically broadens the indications for reconstructive surgery of the elbow. Whereas resurfacing devices may be very effective in rheumatoid arthritis, it is well known that this approach is limited by the amount of bone and the number of soft tissue constraints present [7]. The semiconstrained implant, on the other hand, may be used with equal effectiveness in patients with rheumatoid arthritis [12], post-traumatic arthrosis [13], and revision surgery as well [9]. The enhanced stability provided by this and similar designs is afforded without direct transmission of forces to the bone–cement interface [14].

Right and left specificity is determined by the ulnar stem. The triangular humeral stem is interchangeable. In 1978, the initial design (Coonrad I) was modified to permit 7°–10° of hinge laxity, or toggle, which is consistent with the average laxity of the normal elbow joint (Coonrad II). This change constitutes the semiconstrained designation applied to the device. The effect of this design concept is discussed above (Fig. 1). This implant was designed for use with methylmethacrylate and is manufactured in two sizes: a regular and a small size (15% reduction).

The prosthesis was further modified by the Mayo Clinic in 1981 by adding a band of porous coating of the distal humeral and proximal ulnar stems to permit

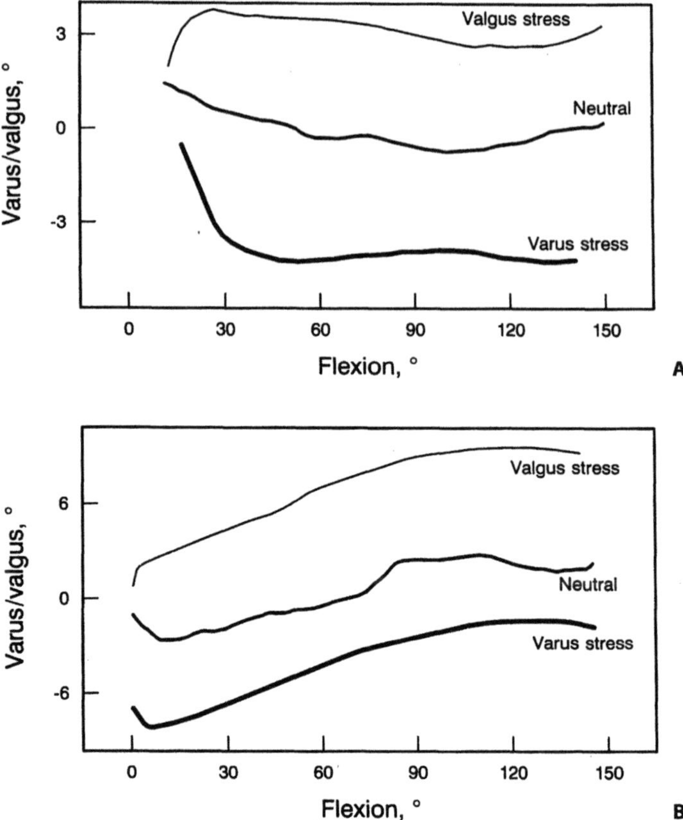

Fig. 1. The kinematics of the normal elbow (**A**) and Coonrad-Morrey total elbow arthroplasty (**B**). The normal elbow follows a neutral path without significant varus/valgus deflection during simulated elbow flexion. Similarly, the Coonrad-Morrey TEA follows a neutral path, though its limits of varus and valgus are greater than those of the normal intact elbow. (Reproduced with permission from Mayo Foundation)

better fixation. An anterior flange was also added to the lower humeral stem, permitting the insertion of a bone graft anteriorly to enhance fixation at the point where maximum stress has been found to occur. This implant is intended to be used with bone cement for both immediate and long-term fixation. The humeral stem comes in 4-, 6-, or 8-inch stem lengths. The 6-inch stem is most commonly used in any practice to ensure adequate mechanical resistance to rotation in the humerus. The 4-inch stem is used in those with rheumatoid arthritis when the shoulder has been or may be replaced with a humeral prosthesis [5]. The 8-inch stem is used with revision procedures needing the device to bypass the prior stem tip [10].

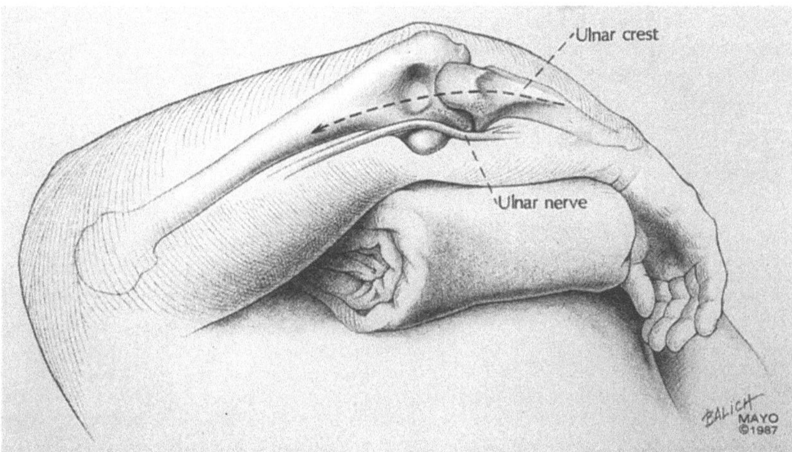

Fig. 2. The patient is placed supine on the operating table. The arm is draped free and brought across the chest. The Mayo (Bryan-Morrey) approach uses a 15-cm incision centered between the medial epicondyle and the tip of the olecranon. (Reproduced with permission from Mayo Foundation)

Surgical Technique

Exposure

The patient is supine with a sandbag under the scapula, and the arm is draped free with a nonsterile tourniquet and brought across the chest (Fig. 2). The Mayo (Bryan-Morrey) approach is used for this procedure [3, 11]. A straight 15-cm incision is centered between the medial epicondyle and the tip of the olecranon. The medial aspect of the triceps is identified, and the ulnar nerve is carefully isolated and translocated using ocular magnification and a bipolar cautery. It is gently protected throughout the remainder of the procedure.

An incision is made over the medial aspect of the proximal ulna, and the ulnar periosteum is elevated along with the forearm fascia. The medial aspect of the triceps is then elevated along with the posterior capsule. The triceps is elevated from the proximal ulna by transecting Sharpey's fibers at the site of insertion. The extensor mechanism, including the anconeus, is reflected laterally, allowing complete exposure of the distal humerus, the proximal ulna, and the radial head. The radial and ulnar collateral ligament complexes are released from the anconeus in those with rheumatoid arthritis.

The tip of the olecranon is removed. The humerus is externally rotated, and the forearm is brought lateral to the humeral shaft.

Fig. 3. An entry hole into the intramedullary canal of the humerus is made in the midportion of the trochlea and a cutting guide is inserted. (Reproduced with permission from Mayo Foundation)

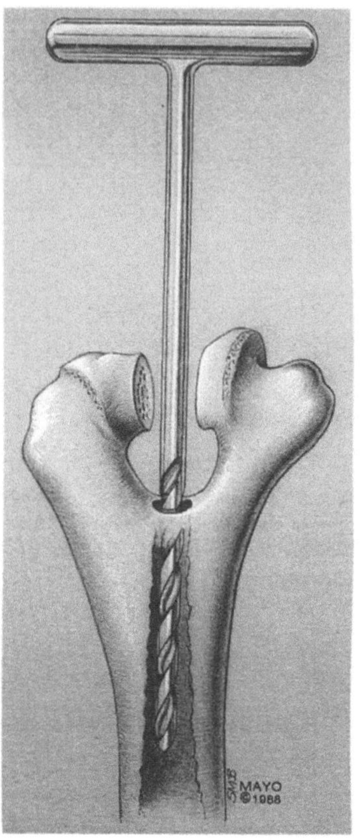

Humeral Preparation

After the ulna and the radius have been rotated out of the way, the midportion of the trochlea is removed with a rongeur or a saw, depending on the softness of the bone. The medullary canal of the humerus is identified by entering it with a rongeur or a burr at the roof of the olecranon fossa. The medullary canal of the humerus is entered with a twist reamer. The medial and lateral aspects of the supracondylar columns should be identified and visualized throughout the preparation of the distal humerus to assure proper alignment and orientation.

The alignment stem is placed down the canal (Fig. 3). The handle is removed and a cutting block is attached, which allows accurate removal of the articular surface of the distal humerus.

The interchangeable side arm of the cutting block is attached laterally to rest on the capitellum in order to provide the appropriate depth of cut. The flat of the template rests on the posterior columns to ensure accurate rotatory alignment. With an oscillating saw, the trochlea is removed according to the dimensions of the appropriate cutting block that corresponds to the sizes of the humeral component.

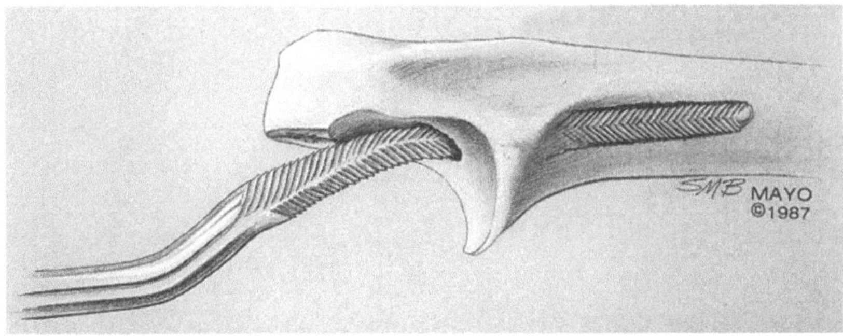

Fig. 4. The appropriate-sized rasp is used to prepare the ulnar canal. Occasionally, the orifice must be opened with a burr. This stage often requires the use of a mallet. (Reproduced with permission from Mayo Foundation)

To avoid fracture, care should be taken not to violate either supracondylar bony column because this may cause a stress riser.

With rheumatoid arthritis, the humerus is easily prepared by a rasp in such a way as to receive the appropriately sized humeral component. In younger patients or in those with post-traumatic conditions, the canal may be tight or the anterior humeral bow may make preparation more difficult.

Ulnar Preparation

The medullary canal of the ulna is identified by using a high-speed burr at about a 45° angle to the base of the coronoid. The tip of the olecranon is removed, notched, or both, to allow identification of the canal by a smaller reamer. An appropriately sized rasp is then used and will generally require the use of a mallet to remove the subchondral bone around the coronoid (Fig. 4).

Implant Insertion

The medullary cavities of both bones are cleansed with a pulsating lavage irrigation system and dried. Insertion of the device may be accomplished by cementing the components individually or coupled. If done individually, cement is injected down the medullary canal of the ulna first with an intramedullary injection system designed to fit even the small canal. The component is inserted distally so that the center of the ulnar component aligns with the projected center of the greater sigmoid fossa, or trochlear notch, of the ulna (Fig. 5).

The cement is then injected down the humeral medullary canal to a depth determined by the length of the humeral stem: 10, 15, or 20 cm. A bone graft is prepared from the excised trochlea or from the iliac crest for revision surgery. The graft should measure about 3–4 mm in thickness and should be about 2 cm in

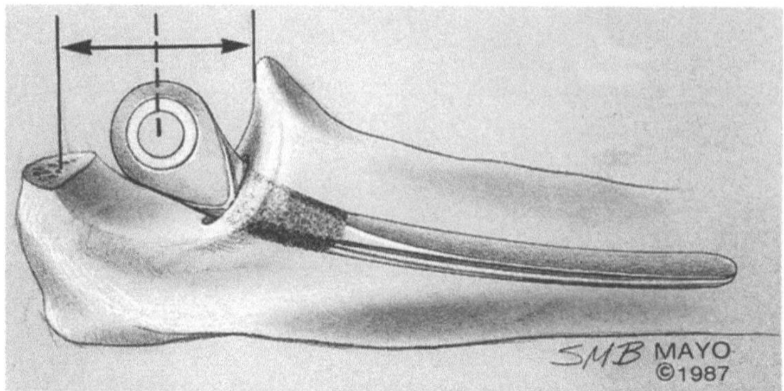

Fig. 5. The ulnar component is inserted so that the center of the bushing is aligned with the center of the trochlear notch of the ulna. (Reproduced with permission from Mayo Foundation)

length and 1.5 cm in width. The bone graft is placed anterior to the anterior cortex of the distal humerus, and the humeral component is inserted down the canal to a point that allows articulation of the device at a level where the bone graft is partially covered by the flange as well (Fig. 6). If the canal is tight, the anterior bow of the humerus is accommodated by placing a slight bow in the humeral stem with the plate bender.

The ulnar component is articulated with the humeral device by placing the axis through the humerus and ulna and securing it with the split-locking ring. After the prosthesis has been coupled, the ulna is placed at a 90° angle, and the

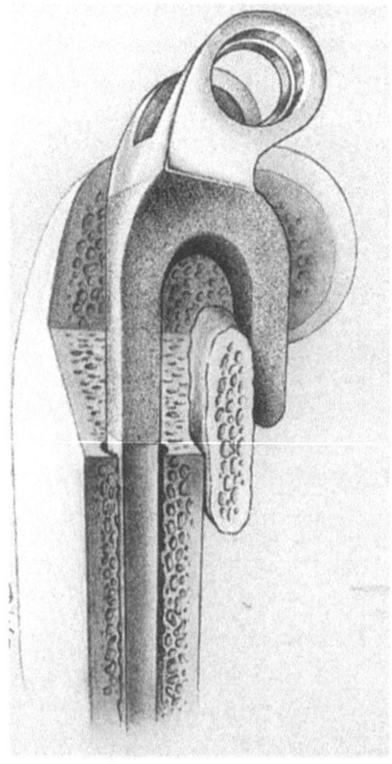

Fig. 6. The humeral component is inserted with a bone graft beneath the anterior flange. The prosthesis must be articulated prior to final insertion of the humeral component. (Reproduced with permission from Mayo Foundation)

humeral component is impacted down the medullary canal. In general, the level of insertion is to a point such that the axis of rotation of the prosthesis is at the level of the normal anatomic axis of rotation. This is approximated when the base of the flange is flushed to the anterior bone of the olecranon fossa and the distal aspect of the humeral component is flush or slightly proximal to the distal aspect of the capitellum.

The cement is permitted to harden with the elbow in full extension. The range of motion is again evaluated, and excess bone and cement anteriorly removed as needed, assuring that none is left anteriorly that might limit flexion.

Triceps

If the triceps has been reflected, it is secured to the ulna with a heavy, nonabsorbable suture. The stitch is criss-crossed through the tendon and the olecranon. An additional transverse suture holds the tendon in place (Fig. 7). Sutures are tied beneath the tendon to avoid a subcutaneous position that can irritate or cause stitch abscess.

Closure

The tourniquet is deflated, and hemostasis is obtained. Two drains are left in the depths and the wound, which is closed in layers. A suture closes the subcutaneous tissue over the translocated ulnar nerve. The rest of the closure is routine.

A compressive dressing is applied with the elbow in full extension and a plaster splint is placed anterior to avoid pressure on the incision line.

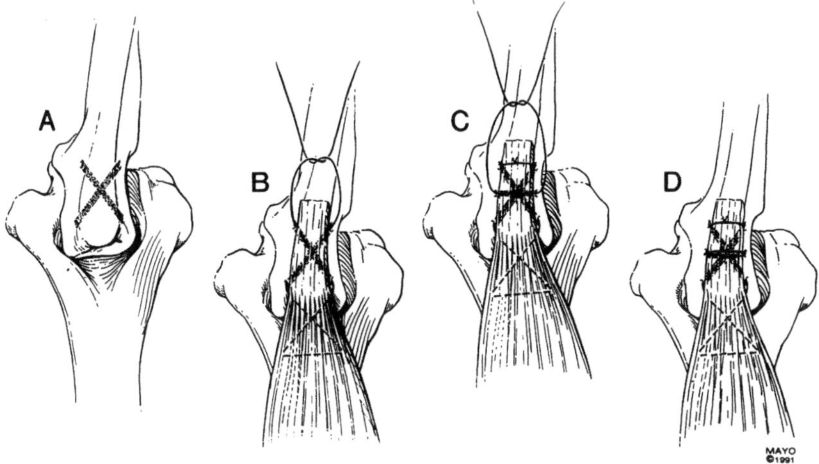

Fig. 7A–D. The triceps is repaired to the olecranon using heavy, nonabsorbable sutures in a Bunnel or modified Kessler technique or a combination of the two techniques. A second transverse stitch is used to hold the triceps down against the bone. (Reproduced with permission from Mayo Foundation)

Postoperative Management

The arm is elevated postoperatively for 2 days with the elbow extended. The drains are removed at approximately 24h, and the compressive dressing is removed on the second or third day after surgery. A light dressing is applied, and elbow flexion and extension is allowed, as tolerated. A collar and cuff are used, and the patient is sent to the occupational therapy unit for activities of daily living. No formal physical therapy is generally required or indicated. Strength exercises are avoided. The patient is advised not to lift more than 1 point over the next 3 months, and we typically recommend that the patient not lift more than 5 points with the operated arm. If a flexion contracture greater than 45° existed before surgery, an extension turnbuckle splint is regularly used at night for 4–12 weeks.

Coonrad Implant

In 1978, the rigid-hinged Coonrad design, used since 1971, was modified to allow approximately 8° of varus/valgus play and 8° of axial rotation. After a very encouraging early experience with this modification, in 1981 a flange and plasma spray were added to the distal humeral component. Since that time, over 250 Coonrad-Morrey implants have been inserted for a variety of problems: rheumatoid arthritis 45%, traumatic arthritis 37%, and revision of prior total elbow arthroplasty 18%. The attractive feature of this particular design is that it includes 4-, 6-, and 8-inch stems. As such, it is used off the shelf for a broad spectrum of conditions. For those with rheumatoid arthritis, a 4-inch stem is sometimes used if a shoulder replacement has been done or is anticipated [5]. The implant is also used in patients with post-traumatic conditions involving variable bone loss as a revision implant or for reconstruction of the flail elbow [1, 4, 13].

Our experience has shown that the semiconstrained implant is a very reliable device for a broad spectrum of elbow pathology. Functionally, the mean arc of motion for the entire group is 26°–130° of flexion, with 64° of pronation and 62° of supination. Pain relief was obtained in 92% of the overall population, and significantly, a dramatic reduction in the complication rate to 15% was observed. Of these, 2% had mechanical loosening and 3% had loosening due to particulate synovitis, which has been eliminated with the more recent design [9]. The 5-year survival for nonseptic failure for all diagnoses for the Coonrad-Morrey implants is about 95%.

Rheumatoid Arthritis

The semiconstrained implant was used primarily for type III and type IV rheumatoid involvement. Our experience with the device using this diagnosis has recently been reported [12]. This degree of involvement often includes the shoulder. Under these circumstances, a 4-inch humeral stem is employed. In this population, the 3-year survival rate of the prosthesis before reoperation was 94%. There have been no revisions for mechanical loosening.

Post-traumatic Arthritis

There is virtually nothing in the literature that focuses on the use of elbow joint replacement for post-traumatic conditions. Hence, we analyzed our experience with 54 consecutive total elbow arthroplasties performed for post-traumatic arthritis [13]. All patients had one of the Coonrad designs:

1. Type I, the early constrained hinge (1971–1978)
2. Type II, the semiconstrained hinge (1978–1981)
3. Type III, the Coonrad-Morrey (1981 to present) Fig. 8;

Preoperatively, 15% of patients had less than 50° of motion, and 13% had flail extremities. With a mean follow-up of over 6 years, ranging from 2 to 14 years, a 76% success rate was noted after the first operation. A revision occurred in 24% and at the time of the last review 85% of the patients are classified as satisfactory without a progressive lucent line or significant pain.

The experience with the current design (Coonray-Morrey) for the post-traumatic condition has recently been updated in 63 patients (unpublished data). A reoperation rate of 13% and a revision rate of only 5% were noted at 3 years. At the time of the last review of the radiographs of the first 26 procedures, four of 26 patients had nonprogressive lucent lines: three about the humerus and one about

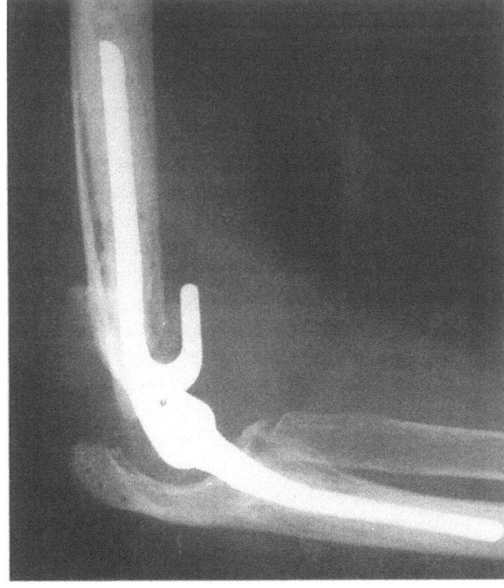

Fig. 8. Coonrad-Morrey total elbow arthroplasty in place 5 years postoperatively with no radiographic evidence of loosening. The bone graft beneath the anterior flange has been incorporated and the underlying distal humeral bone remodeled. (Reproduced with permission from Mayo Foundation)

the ulnar component. Overall, a satisfactory rate of over 90% was present in this difficult group of patients with follow-up of 1–10 years.

Conclusion

The reported experience with the semiconstrained total joint replacement is dramatically and significantly better than that reported for the more constrained devices. Overall, the loose-hinged semiconstrained implants provide a significant enhancement of the options and indications for the use of joint replacement. In our experience, in rheumatoid patients, the reliability is comparable to that of the resurfacing implant. Additional time is required before the full impact of these studies is known. The current data allow cautious optimism with regard to the use of semiconstrained elbow joint replacement.

References

1. Bell S, Gschwend N, Steiger U (1986) Arthroplasty of the elbow. Experience with the mark III GSB prosthesis. Aust NZ J Surg 56:823–827
2. Brumfield RH, Kuschner SH, Gellman H, Redix L, Stevenson DV (1990) Total elbow arthroplasty. J Arthr 5:359–363
3. Bryan RS, Morrey BF (1982) Extensive posterior exposure of the elbow: a triceps-sparing approach. Clin Orthop 166:188–192
4. Davis RF, Weiland AJ, Hungerford SD, Moore JR, Volenec-Dowling S (1982) Nonconstrained total elbow arthroplasty. Clin Orthop 171:156–160
5. Friedman RJ, Ewald FC (1987) Arthroplasty of the ipsilateral shoulder and elbow in patients who have rheumatoid arthritis. J Bone Joint Surg 69-A:661–666
6. Gschwend N, Loehr J, Ivosevic-Radovanovic D, Scheier H, Munzinger U (1988) Semiconstrained elbow prostheses with special reference to the GSB III prosthesis. Clin Orthop 232:104–111
7. Lindscheid RL (1993) Resurfacing elbow replacement arthroplasty: rationale, technique, and results. In: Morrey BF (ed) The elbow and its disorders. Saunders, Philadelphia, pp 638–647
8. Madsen F, Gudmundson GH, Søjbjerg JO, Sneppen O (1989) The pritchard mark II elbow prosthesis in rheumatoid arthritis. Acta Orthop Scand 60:249–253
9. Morrey BF (1991) Semi-constrained total elbow arthroplasty. In: Morrey BF (ed) Joint replacement arthroplasty. Churchill Livingstone, New York
10. Morrey BF (1993) Revision of failed total elbow arthroplasty. In: Morrey BF (ed) The elbow and its disorders. Saunders, Philadelphia, pp 676–689
11. Morrey BF (1993) Surgical exposures of the elbow. In: Morrey BF (ed) The elbow and its disorders. Saunders, Philadelphia, pp 139–166
12. Morrey BF, Adams RA (1992) Semiconstrained arthroplasty for the treatment of rheumatoid arthritis of the elbow. J Bone Joint Surg 74-A:479–490
13. Morrey BF, Adams RA, Bryan RS (1991) Total replacement for post-traumatic arthritis of the elbow. J Bone Joint Surg 73-B:607–612
14. O'Driscoll SW, An K-N, Korinek S, Morrey BF (1992) Kinematics of semi-constrained total elbow arthroplasty. J Bone Joint Surg 74-B:297–299

The Norway Elbow System*

F. Risung

Design

The Norway elbow is a long-stemmed, unconstrained elbow prosthesis, produced in four different humeral sizes and three different ulnar sizes for the right and left sides. All sizes have an identical joint part, which permits full interchangeability of humeral and ulnar components (Fig. 1).

The humeral component carries a rotating polyethylene bobbin on a slanting axle screw, corresponding to the normal carrying angle of the elbow. The ulnar component has a claw-like joint part gripping loosely around the humeral bobbin, giving an inbuilt freedom of toggle of approximately 6° (Fig. 2) [4].

It is not a snap-fit joint; the collateral ligaments must be stretched 8 mm during the final reduction of the prosthesis, as stability is dependent on intact and functioning collateral ligaments and tendons. The description of the prosthesis by Morrey [3] as a snap-fit joint is not accurate in this respect.

That the prosthesis really functions as an unconstrained prosthesis and can replicate the normal biomechanics of the elbow has been showed by King et al. [1].

The prosthesis allows a much greater range of motion than the normal elbow and depends on functioning ligaments and tendons for stability (Fig. 3). If the ligamental support is temporarily insufficient, an optional locking ring may be applied (Fig. 2). This constraining ring is not intended as an articulation, but merely to act as a check-rein for preventing dislocation of the prosthesis.

Materials

The prosthesis is machined from certified materials of medical-grade wrought titanium alloy (Ti-6AI-4Va) and HD-HMW polyethylene. All components of the prosthesis may be sterilized by autoclaving (121°C), including the polyethylene bobbin (if protected from pressure from other items while hot). The prosthesis will be commercially available preassembled and sterile.

---

*The Norway elbow was designed by F. Risung in collaboration with J. Teigland and J. Pahle and is manufactured by Brødrene Johnsen AS, 1400 Ski, Norway.

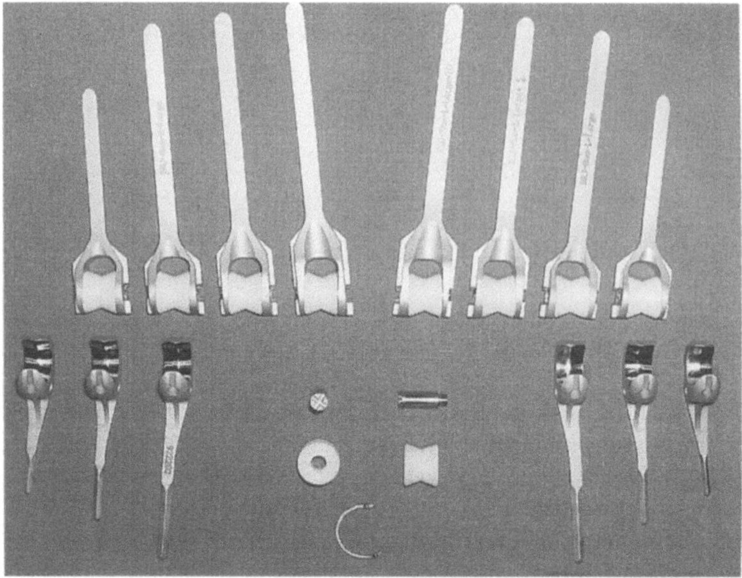

Fig. 1. The complete set of implants for the right and left elbow. The lower center shows the axle screw, the bobbin, and the optional semiconstraining clip

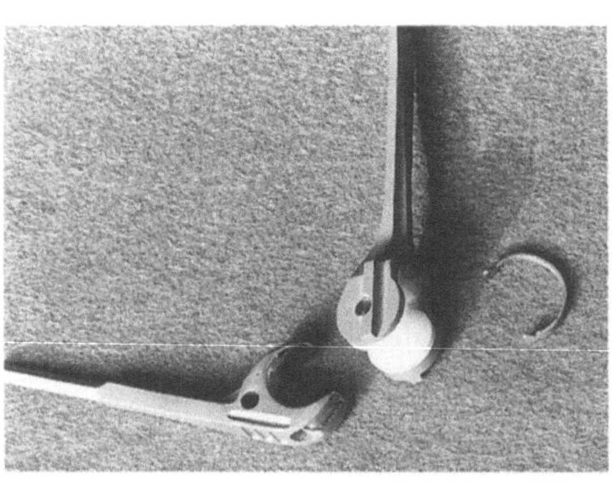

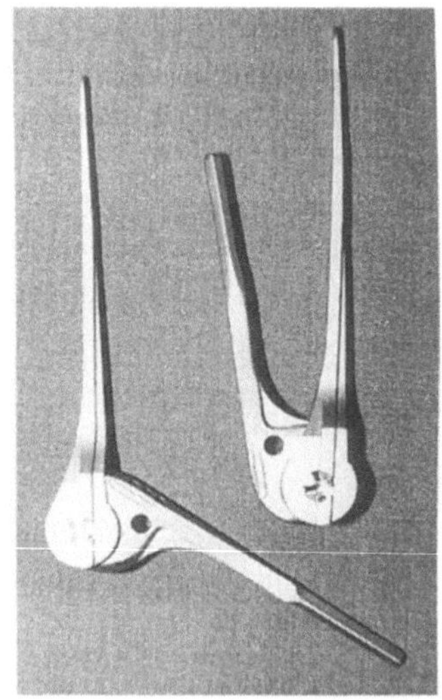

Fig. 2. Details of the loose claw-like joint. The semiconstraining ring may be clipped around the bobbin and clicked into grooves on the ulnar component in cases with insufficient ligaments under repair. Note the long side-flanges of the humeral component
Fig. 3. Side view of the assembled prosthesis. *Left*, Maximum hyperextension of more than 45°. *Right*, Maximum flexion of 175°. Range of motion is limited only by the soft tissues and the ligaments

Indications

The primary indication is destructive rheumatoid arthritis. The prosthesis can also be used for severe arthrosis and selected cases of traumatic disorders.

Contraindications

Common medical contraindications include inadequate bony or ligamentous support and inadequate soft tissue covering.

Surgical Procedure

We perform the operation through a posterior triceps-splitting incision, preserving the continuity of the lateral and long heads of the muscle, the tendon, and the fascia on both sides of the incision. The radial head is always resected. The ulnar nerve is antepositioned only if necessary. All ligaments are carefully spared, and a minimum of bone resection is necessary (20 mm of the central part of the trochlea humeri and a 90° wedge of the proximal ulna).

Special tools are provided for reaming the bones and handling the implants (Fig. 4). After testing the ligaments for stability and adequate laxity for reduction

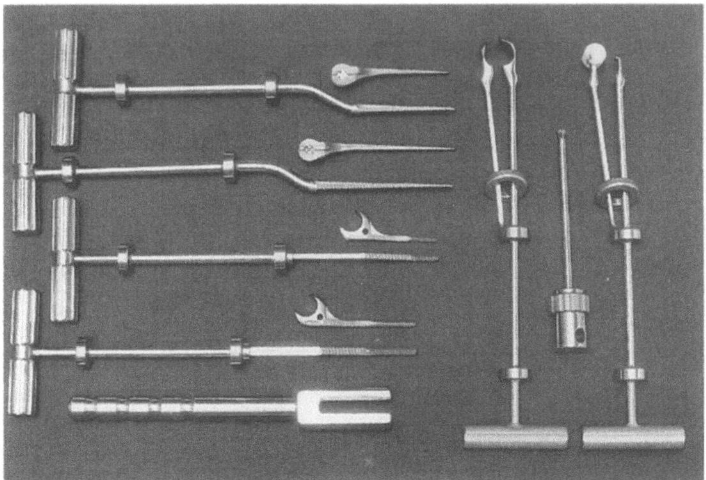

Fig. 4. The complete set of special instruments for the prosthesis. *Left* (*from top*), small and large humeral rasps, small and large ulnar rasps, and the slotted hammer, which can be used on all instruments. *Center*, trial components shown with their corresponding rasps. *Right*, introducer/extractor for the humeral component, screwdriver for axle screw, and introducer/extractor for the ulnar component

of the prosthesis, both components are cemented with standard PMMA (Palacos with gentamicin). The fixation of the humeral component is enhanced by long side-flanges on both sides of the component, past the joint axis of rotation.

Total Case Material

More than 300 prostheses have been used in our two clinics in Oslo and Skien from August 1982 until January 1994, with a mean observation time of 4.2 years. A total of 116 operations were performed more than 5 years ago. Several other hospitals have now also started using this prosthesis, and others are following.

The Oslo cases (200 prostheses) were not followed with a prospective protocol and were reviewed retrospectively during 1994; they cannot presently be accounted for.

The 100 prostheses in Skien have been followed prospectively, with regular follow-ups after 3, 6, and 12 months and annually thereafter. A full report on the present results concerning these patients was given at the congress on the elbow in Düsseldorf (March 1994).

Skien Case Material

A total of 100 prostheses were used in 71 patients; 29 had bilateral implants, and only 42 prostheses were unilateral. All patients suffered from severe destructive rheumatoid arthritis (Larsen-Dale-Eeg grade 4 or 5 or worse).

Ten patients carrying 13 prostheses died during the program; one of these prostheses was removed early due to deep infection. No other prostheses have been removed in any of the Skien cases.

The mean observation time is 3.8 years (0.2–7.0 years); 62 prostheses have had more than 3 years observation time, and 30 prostheses more than 5 years observation time.

Results

Almost complete pain relief, good functional improvement, and a modest gain in range of motion is achieved (as with most elbow prostheses). The mean gain in flexion/extension, after more than 5 years, is 23.2°, the mean reduction of flexion contracture being 10°. The mean gain in rotation of the forearm is 21.3°.

Complications

Very few serious complications have occurred. As already mentioned, only one of the 100 prostheses has been removed. Only one aseptic loosening has occurred after 7 years of symptom-free use. This prosthesis has so far been successfully exchanged with a new prosthesis.

Two very early dislocations of the prosthetic joint have occurred, both in rheumatic patients who also had badly healed comminuted fractures of the distal humerus. These dislocations were due to insufficient collateral ligaments. One elbow was successfully revised with osteosynthesis of the epicondyles and has since been stable for 3 years. The other elbow dislocated repeatedly despite several attempts at revision. It was ultimately infected, and the prosthesis had to be removed.

Two axle screws have loosened due to sloppy primary fastening within the first ten operations before this was recognized as a possible hazard. The first (operation no. 10) was seen immediately after the implantation (see "Salvation Procedure" below), and the other was identified on radiographs after 6 years, but the patient is still symptom free and the elbow is functioning well.

One case of bilateral epicondylar fractures of the humerus occurred 2 months after the procedure, probably due to excessively tight fitting of the humeral component (excessively narrow resection). Two other patients sustained bilateral epicondylar humeral fractures, one preoperatively when an anesthetized osteoporotic and contracted elbow was extended, the other during a hasty reduction of the joint after a momentary cardiac arrest. No fractures have occurred directly related to the saw cuts or the resection of the humerus.

We have experienced ten cases of ulnar nerve affections; one was a direct ulnar nerve lesion, two needed decompression of the nerve, and the other were transitory.

Seven patients have a weakened triceps function. Three patients had periarticular extruded cement, one cement lump had to be removed, and the other patients are symptom free.

Seven patients had superficial infections cured by antibiotics. Two had deep infections of the joint; in one of these the prosthesis had to be removed, as described above, and the other is described below.

Salvation Procedure

Patient no. 10, a 75.6-year-old man with severely destructive arthritis, had a primary loose axle screw, no pain, and good function. The patient was frail and had fragile skin from long-term corticoid therapy. We refrained from revision until 3 years after the operation he sustained a hematogenous deep infection in the elbow joint after a pneumonia. He was referred to us with an open fistula onto the prosthesis after incision and evacuation of pus containing pneumococci.

The elbow was revised with a wide opening of the scar and excision of the fistula. There was surprisingly little metallosis. We were able to drill through the epicondyles and extract the loose axle screw, after which the ulna with the bobbin could slide backwards and out of the humeral component. The joint was cleaned out, and a new bobbin was inserted. The elbow was then replaced and a new axle screw inserted. The joint was closed in layers and healed promptly under antibiotic therapy. The elbow was pain free and functioning well for 2 years after the revision, when the patient died from heart failure and a probable lung cancer.

This experience shows that the axle bolt and the bobbin can both be exchanged with new parts if necessary, particularly if excessive wear of the bobbin should occur in the future.

The locking ring has not yet been used in a patient. It was designed as a result of the two dislocated prostheses that we experienced with the patients with distal humerus fractures and insufficient collateral ligament support. The dislocations in these cases might have been avoided if this semiconstraining device had been available at that time.

The locking ring may be applied at any stage of the operation if the ligamental support should be insufficient. The locking ring may also be removed if no longer required.

Titanium Alloy

This prosthesis was designed in 1976, and the very best biocompatible material at that time, titanium alloy, was chosen for the metal parts, combined with ultrahigh molecular weight, high-density polyethylene for the bobbin [2].

During the 12 years that this prosthesis has been used, we have not experienced any clinical adverse effects of this combination of materials.

In recent years several reports have been published [5] in which the biocompatibility of titanium alloy has been questioned due to heavy metallosis. However, this issue is controversial, and metallosis, with or without inflammation, occurs even in prostheses made of stainless steel or chrome-cobalt alloys.

We have revised two of our prostheses and also been able to retrieve another two prostheses at autopsy several years after the implantation. In these cases we have observed varying degrees of metallosis, from very mild to quite severe. In the latter case (revision after 7 years), the tissues were microscopically discolored with extracellular brownish deposits of foreign material, as well as spindle-shaped crystalline material of uncertain origin inside multinuclear foreign body cells. This case otherwise showed very little inflammatory reaction. Another case, retrieved after 3 years, showed considerable discoloration from hemosiderin as well as some deposits of extracellular brownish particles and some inflammatory reaction. None of these patients had any clinical synovitis or pain in the elbow prior to retrieval. None of our patients have shown any signs of recurring synovitis in the operated elbow joints.

The clinical implications of these findings are uncertain. We are preparing for nitrogen ion implantation on the joint surfaces of the metal components to improve the wear characteristics of the titanium alloy [6]. We have found no sincere justification for changing the materials in the prosthesis.

References

1. King GJW, Itoi E, Risung F, Niebur GL, Morrey BF, An K-N (1993) Kinematics and stability of the Norway elbow. A cadaveric study. Acta Orthop Scand 64(6):657–663
2. Lemons JE (1991) Metallic alloys. In: Morrey BF (ed) Joint replacement arthroplasty. Churchill Livingstone, New York, pp 18–21
3. Morrey BF (1993) The elbow and its disorders. Saunders, Philadelphia, p 659
4. Risung F (1991) Characteristics, design and preliminary results of the «Norway elbow system». Rheumatology 15:68–72
5. Williams D (1994) The capricious nature of biocompatibility. Medical device technology. Advanstar Communications, Chester, pp 8–11
6. Shioshansi P (1990) Improving the properties of titanium alloys by ion implantation. J Materials, pp 30–31

Cementless or Hybrid Total Elbow Arthroplasty – A Study of Interim Clinical Results and Specific Complications

H. Kudo

In 1988 the type-4 prosthesis (Fig. 1) was developed with the aim of fixing the prosthesis without cement. The humeral component was made of titanium alloy, and a porous coated stem was attached to the condylar portion. The ulnar component was made of high-density polyethylene, and for the first 2 years an all-polyethylene component was used. However, at the end of 1989 the ulnar component was changed to the present version with a metal back support. The purpose of this modification was so that it may be used not only with, but also without cement in suitable cases.

The type-4 prosthesis is nonlinked and nonconstrained, and only minimal bone resection is needed because surface replacement is a fundamental concept with this prosthesis. In general, the two components do not need cement for their fixation. The geometry of the articular surface of both components is of monofacet shape with a small clearance between them, allowing slight mediolateral movement during the elbow movement.

The present series include 32 elbows (ankylosis, $n = 3$; stiff elbow, $n = 12$; unstable elbow, $n = 17$) in 26 patients with rheumatoid arthritis which were operated on during a 2-year period from 1988 to 1990. The average follow-up was 4 years and 2 months (range, 3 years and 3 months to 5 years and 6 months). The humeral component was fixed without cement in all 32 elbows, while the ulnar component was fixed without cement in only four elbows. Thus in 28 elbows, fixation was performed by the hybrid method, and in the remaining four elbows completely cementless fixation was performed.

The key points of the operative technique are as follows:

1. Campbell's posterior approach is routinely used.
2. In most cases the medial collateral ligament is released.
3. The radial head is resected and no attempt is made to replace it.
4. The ulnar nerve is extensively released in the first stage of the operation and is transferred anteriorly at the end of the operation.
5. As many chips as possible of autogenous bone graft are used to pack the empty space inside the condylar portion of the humeral component.
6. Cementless fixation should be possible in 95% of cases for the humeral component, while for the ulnar component it should be possible in around 50% of cases.

Fig. 1. The type-4 prosthesis

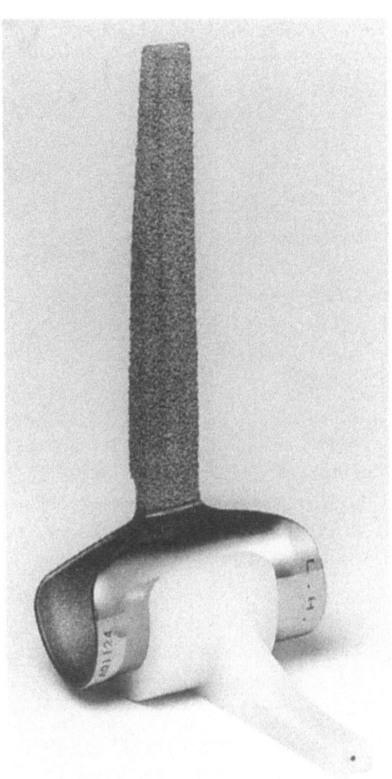

A modified version of Morrey's criteria was used for assessment of the overall results (Table 1). In this criteria an elbow which gains 75 or more points is rated as good. An elbow which gains 50–74 points is rated fair, and less than 50 points, poor.

The overall results were as follows: five elbows showed poor results because of the fracture at the base of the stem of the humeral component and all five needed revision. Two elbows were rated fair (acceptable), and 25 were rated good (satisfactory). Regarding the range of motion, flexion and forearm rotation were improved significantly after operation, while the flexion contracture was not improved (Table 2).

The results of the radiographic assement were as follows: with the humeral component, a translucent line around the stem was not seen in any of the 32 elbows, i.e., successful biologic fixation of the stem was achieved in all elbows. Mild subsidence of the humeral component was seen in only one elbow.

The biggest problem was the occurrence of variable degrees of osteolysis of the distal portion of the humeral condyles. Severe osteolysis was seen in six elbows, and out of these six elbows, five were complicated by fracture of the stem. There was moderate osteolysis in three elbows, mild osteolysis in 18, and no osteolysis in five. With the ulnar component, a translucent line around the cement mass was seen in two out of 28 cemented ulnar components. A translucent line in the proximal portion only was found in seven elbows, and no line was found in 19.

Table 1. Classification of results

Criteria	Points
Pain	
None	60
Mild to occasional; no medication	40
Moderate to occasional; medication; activity limited	20
Severe to incapacitating	0
Motion: arc of extension/flexion	
$\geq 90°$	30
$60°–89°$	20
$30°–59°$	10
$<30°$	0
Stability: effect on function of the elbow	
None or mild (does not limit activity)	10
Moderate (impairs certain functions)	5
Severe (markedly limits activity)	0
Classification of result, based on total points	
Good (satisfactory)	≥ 75
Fair (acceptable)	50–74
Poor (unsatisfactory)[a]	<50

[a] Regardless of the point score, an ankylosed elbow is rated as poor.

Table 2. Average range of motion

	Preoperative	Postoperative
Flexion	106	131
Extension	38	41
Supination	40	61
Pronation	39	46

Regarding the four ulnar components which were fixed without cement, only one showed a thin translucent line around the stem, but no migration of the component was seen.

Figure 2 shows a radiograph of moderate osteolysis. Many bone trabeculae can be seen running toward the stem. Figure 3 shows an X-ray taken soon after fracture of the stem. The presence of fine cracks at the junctional portion and posterior inclination of the condylar portion relative to the stem can be seen.

At the time of revision difficulty was encountered in extracting the stem. It was necessary to cut out all the adhering bone around the stem before retrieval of the stem. Another finding at revision was dark gray or black staining of the soft tissue within the joint. The histology of the soft tissue shows the presence of many black particles of metal debris and inflammatory response with marked histiocytic infiltration (Fig. 4). Figure 5 is a picture of one of the retrieved prostheses. It can be seen that there is a great deal of bone sticking to the stem

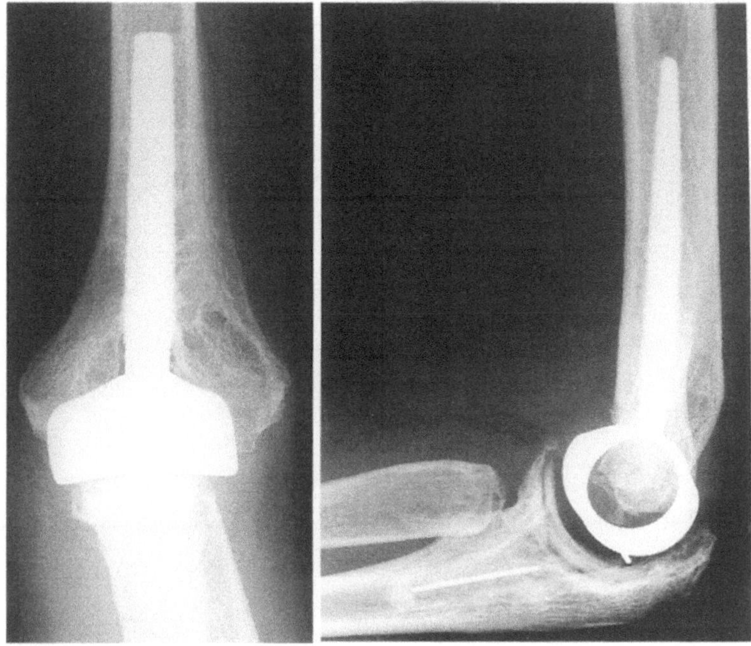

Fig. 2a,b. Moderate osteolysis. Note the trabeculae running towards the stem

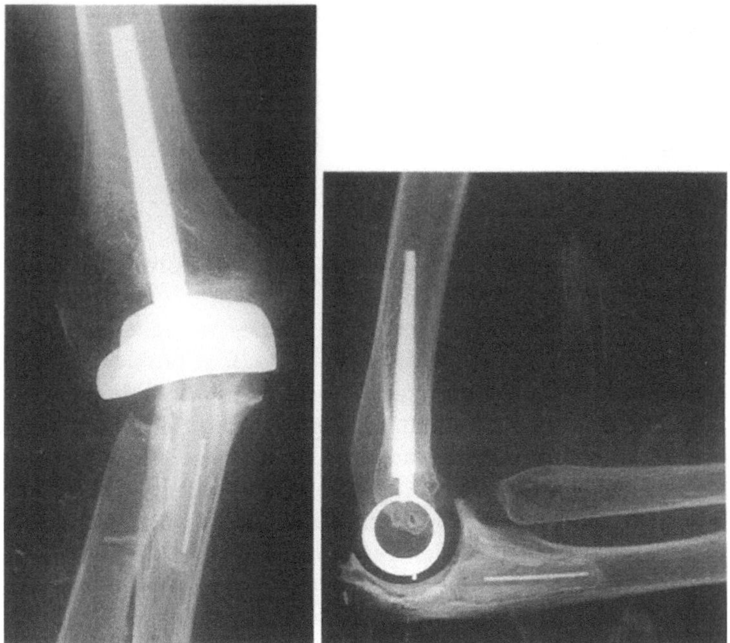

Fig. 3a,b. X-ray taken soon after fracture of the stem

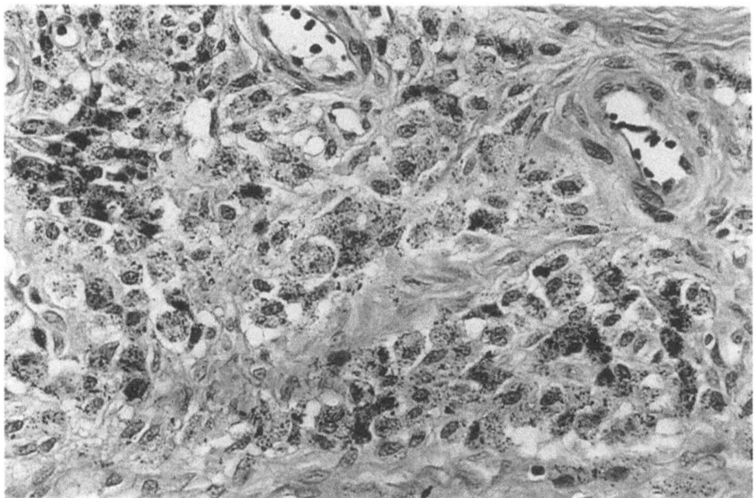

Fig. 4. Metal debris (*black particles*) and inflammatory response with marked histiocytic infiltration

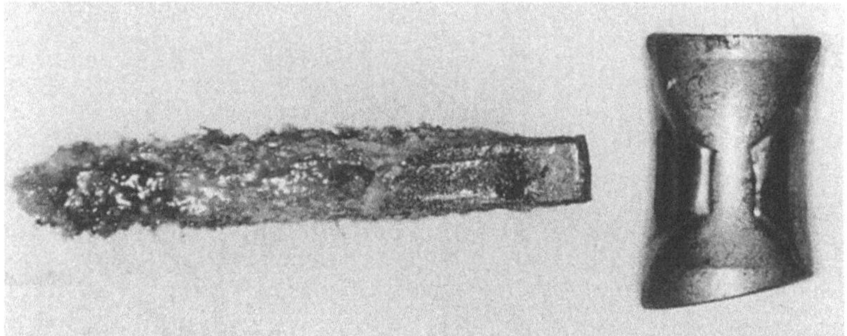

Fig. 5. Retrieved prosthesis

and also that some surface area of the condylar portion looks burnished by wear of the metal.

Through the experience of this series we have learned that there are two problems with the type-4 prosthesis. The first problem concerns titanium alloy, which is used for the humeral component: first, this metal may wear when used in a non-weight-bearing joint such as the elbow and may lead to metallosis, and subsequent histiocytic reactions cause osteolysis of the humeral condyles and ultimately give rise to loss of bony support to the condylar portion; second, excellent biocompatibility of this metal make it possible to achieve secure biologic fixation of the stem in high percentages of cases, so in the presence of osteolysis of the humeral condyles subsidence of the humeral component does not occur, leaving the condylar portion without any bony support. This situation induces stress concentration at the base of the stem and ultimately leads to fatigue fracture.

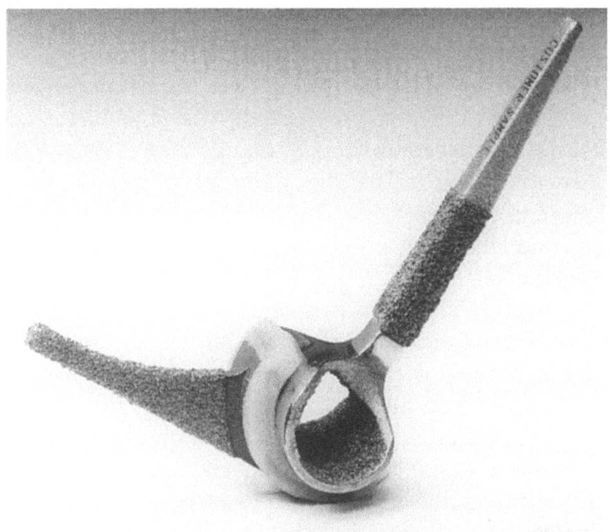

Fig. 6. The type-5 prosthesis

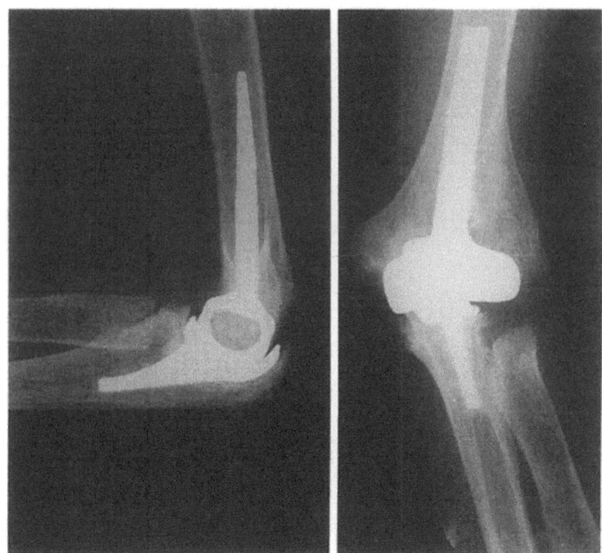

Fig. 7. Type-5 prosthesis in situ 1 year after operation

The second problem is the design of the humeral component; there is a notch posteriorly at the base of the stem, and this notch is made to accept the posterior lip of the ulnar component at the position of full extension. It is possible that this notch constitutes a cause of mechanical weakness and makes it liable to fracture.

What, then, are the solutions to these problems? We first noticed the problem of metal wear with this prosthesis in 1990; in 1991 we introduced the ion implantation process in order to improve the properties of the bearing surface in this respect. We hoped to prevent metallosis and subsequent osteolysis by this method. However, we were concerned that this may not be a good enough solution, and we thought a more radical change might be needed. Thus, at the beginning of 1993 we began to use a humeral component made of cobalt-chromium alloy (type 5); in this new version, a posterior notch was removed and this portion was reinforced with thick metal.

Figure 6 shows the new version (type 5). It can be seen that the base of the stem is reinforced and looks mechanically strong. In addition, the area of porous coating on the stem is reduced to the proximal half. Figure 7 shows the type-5 prosthesis in situ 1 year after the operation.

In conclusion, it has been found that there are two problems with the type-4 prosthesis: tissue metallosis and subsequent osteolysis, and mechanical weakness at the base of the stem of the humeral component. It has also been found that both components of this prosthesis can successfully be fixed without cement even in the osteopenic bone of patients with rheumatoid arthritis. We are now very hopeful that the new version (type 5) will eliminate these problems and achieve long-term success.

Early Results with the Capitellocondylar Total Elbow Prosthesis in Rheumatoid Arthritis

P. Ljung and U. Rydholm

Introduction

The capitellocondylar elbow is a chrome–cobalt resurfacing prosthesis with short intramedullary stems, intended for cemented use (Fig. 1). It is available in one regular size with a thin or regular-sized stem on the ulnar component and one 15% oversized model. Four-, 6- or 9-mm-thick polyethylene is available for the regular-sized ulnar component and 4-, 7- or 10-mm polyethylene for the oversized ulnar component. The medullary fixation stem on the humeral component is available in a 5°, 10°, 15°, or 20° valgus angle. We have so far only used the regular-sized humeral component with 5° stem angle and most often an ulnar component with the thin intramedullar stem. It is a true resurfacing type of prosthesis, and only a very small amount of bone has to be removed (Fig. 2), leaving a reasonable chance for revision.

The capitellocondylar prosthesis has been in clinical use since 1974 and the design remains essentially unchanged. Low revision rates have been reported in long-term follow-ups [1, 3, 4]. In Lund, the capitellocondylar elbow has been used since 1989. Indications for surgery have primarily been relief of pain and secondarily restoration of a functional range of motion in patients with rheumatoid arthritis.

Patients and Methods

Forty-two patients (four men, 38 women) with a median age of 62 years (range, 25–80 years) underwent 50 total elbow replacements with the capitellocondylar elbow prosthesis at the Department of Orthopedics in Lund. Thirty-seven patients had rheumatoid arthritis and five had juvenile chronic arthritis with a mean disease duration of 22 years. All elbows were followed prospectively at 4 months and then yearly. Median follow-up was 30 months (range, 12–59 months).

The radiographs were classified according to Larsen-Dale-Ek. Two thirds of the elbows were grade 4 or 5.

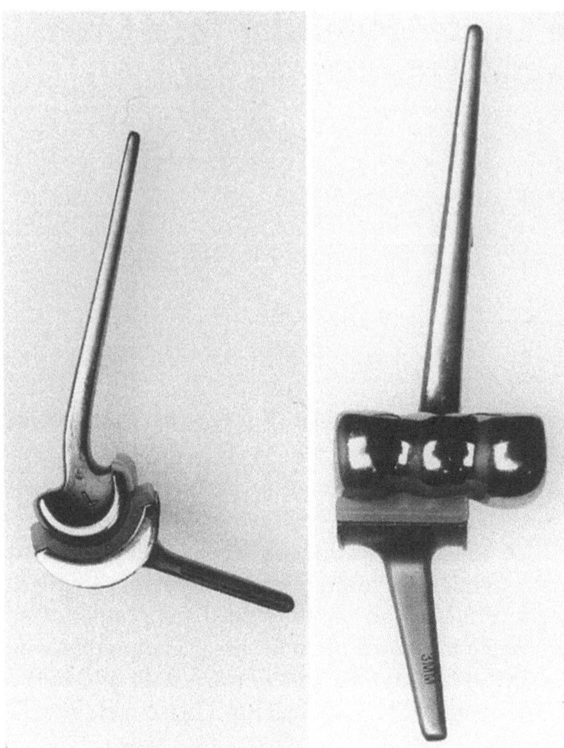

Fig. 1a,b. The capitellocondylar prosthesis with 5° valgus angulation of the humeral component. The ulnar component comes with three different thicknesses of the polyethylene (4, 5, and 9 mm). a Lateral view. b Frontal view

Surgical Technique

The lateral, expanded Kocher approach [2] was used. The radial collateral ligament is cut at its condylar insertion and reflected with the capsule. After synovectomy, removal of the radial head, and subperiostal release of the radial part of the ulnar insertion of the triceps tendon, the joint is dislocated with the medial collateral ligament acting as a hinge. The humerus is then prepared with chisels, rasps, and dental burrs. Only a minor amount of bone has to be removed, especially in joints with preoperative bone loss, which is often most pronounced on the ulnar side of the distal humerus. It is important to restore the center of rotation, which means that the humeral component should be placed in 5° of internal rotation relative to an imaginary line between the two condyles, i.e., the center of the capitellum is placed approximately 1 cm anterior to the lateral condyle. The trochlear notch of the ulna is then prepared with dental burrs or a larger cylindrical burr. It is important to place the ulnar component in neutral rotation, and the correct longitudinal placement is determined by the posterior edge of the component being placed even with the tip of the olecranon. In the case of severe bone loss of the ulna, a thicker polyethylene component is choosen. The articulation is then checked

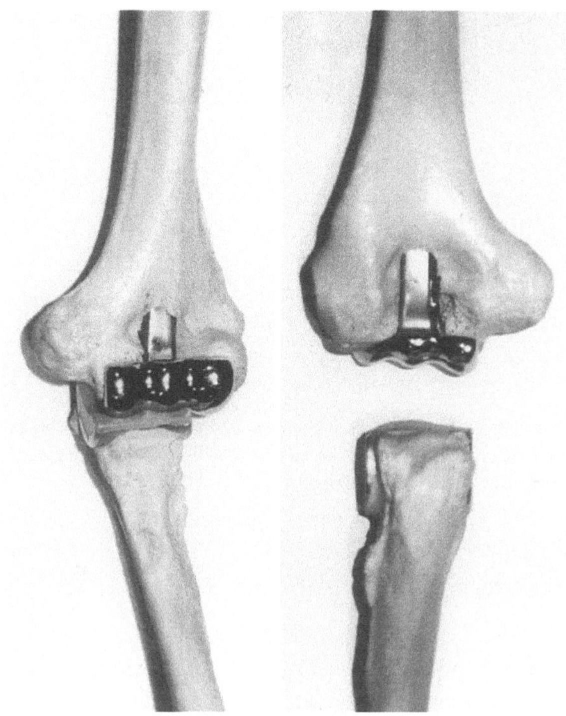

Fig. 2a,b. The prosthesis is a resurfacing type of prosthesis with intramedullary stems to enhance fixation. Note the small amount of humeral intercondylar bone that has to be removed. **a** Anterior view. **b** Posterior view

with the trial components. If it is too loose, a thicker ulnar component is choosen. If it opens up laterally due to a tight medial collateral ligament, more bone is removed from the distal humerus and the rotation or the ulnar component checked. When the trial components track smoothly through the whole range of motion, the definite components are cemented with Palacos with gentamicin. The bone is prepared with high-pressure irrigation and after placement of bony or plastic intramedullary plugs the bone cement is introduced by a cement gun.

Postoperative Regime

From the beginning of this series, the elbows were immobilized for 5 days. The postoperative regime was altered for the remainder of the elbows, which were immobilized for 12 days. A hinged brace (Fig. 3) permitting flexion, extension, and pronation, but preventing supination to save the reinserted radial collateral ligament, was then used for another 4 weeks.

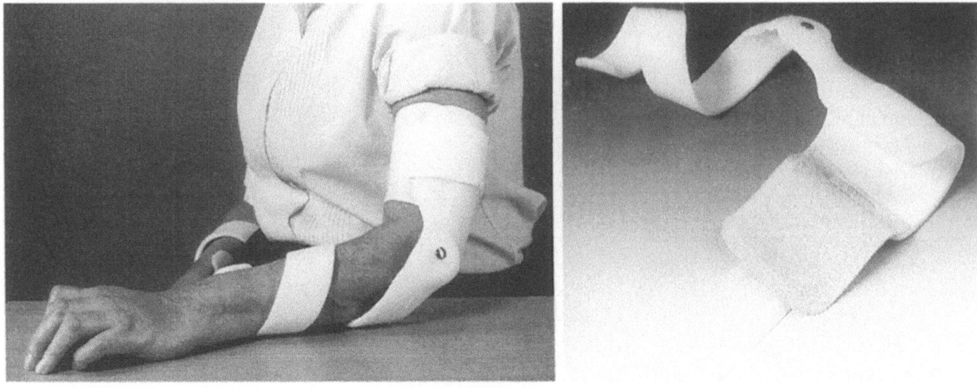

Fig. 3a,b. The hinged brace used during rehabilitation for 6 weeks. **a** It is easy to put on for a patient with rheumatoid destruction of the hands. **b** It prevents varus/valgus forces and supination, while permitting full flexion/extension

Results

Major complications were a traumatic wound rupture and prosthetic dislocation in a patient who fell on her arm in the immediate postoperative course and one late hematogenous infection in a patient with rheumatoid vasculitis. Minor complications were delayed wound healing in two elbows, transient postoperative ulnar nerve palsy in 11 elbows, persistent in three elbows, and lateral translocation of the ulnar component in one elbow. Two secondary wound sutures were performed. Both wounds healed without signs of infection. The ulnar nerve was decompressed in four elbows with ulnar nerve palsy. Ulnar nerve function was fully restituted in three and partly in one of these elbows. The elbow with traumatic prosthetic dislocation was reoperated with lateral collateral ligament reconstruction twice. Stability and function is now good. The prosthesis of the elbow with hematogenous infection was removed.

Pain relief was excellent. Pain on motion and at rest was estimated from a visual analogue scale from 0 to 9. Preoperatively, pain on motion was on average 5, and postoperatively it was 0. Pain at rest was on average 3 preoperatively and 0 postoperatively. There was a gain in range of motion in both extension/flexion and supination/pronation. Mean extension increased from −43° to −35°, while mean flexion increased from 129° to 145°. The range of motion thus increased from a mean of 121° to 135°. All 49 elbows with retained prostheses were stable at follow-up 1 year postoperatively.

Radiographic evaluation revealed no complete radiolucencies (Fig. 4). An incomplete radiolucent zone was found around the cement of one humeral component in a patient without clinical symptoms. A lateral translocation of one ulnar component was found in an elbow without clinical signs or symptoms of instability.

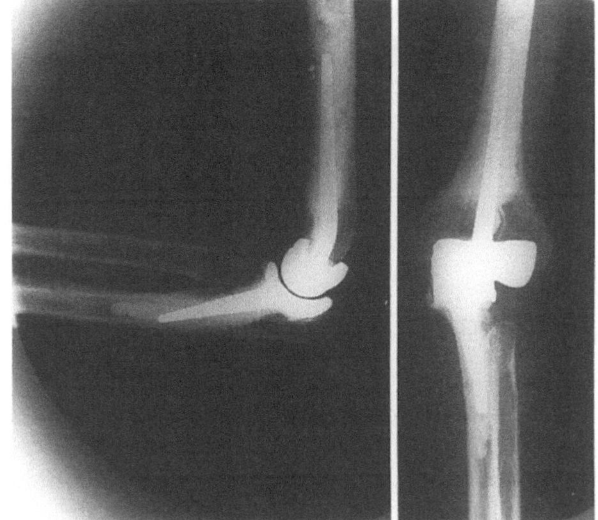

Fig. 4a,b. Radiographs of a capitellocondylar prosthesis 2 years after operation. **a** Correct positioning with a restored center of rotation. **b** No radiolucent lines

Concluding Remarks

We conclude that the early results with the capitellocondylar total elbow in rheumatoid arthritis are excellent. Severe complications are uncommon, but transient postoperative ulnar nerve palsy if frequent.

References

1. Ewald FC, Simmons ED, Sullivan JA, Thomas WH, Scott RD, Poss R, Thornhill TS, Sledge CB (1993) Capitellocondylar total elbow replacement in rheumatoid arthritis. J Bone Joint Surg 75-A:498–507
2. Morrey BF (ed) (1994) The elbow. Master techniques in orthopaedic surgery. Raven, New York
3. Ruth JT, Wilde AH (1991) Capitellocondylar total elbow replacement, a long term follow-up study. Orthop Trans 15:22
4. Weiland AJ, Weiss APC, Wills RP, Moore JR (1989) Capitellocondylar total elbow replacement. A long-term follow-up study. J Bone Joint Surg 71-A:217–222

Complications After Total Elbow Arthroplasty – Unusual Solutions to Different Situations

A. Sosna, I. Landor, and M. Richtr

Introduction

Total elbow arthroplasty has been routinely performed at the Orthopedic Clinic of the University of Prague since 1987. We use the Souter-Strathclyde total elbow replacement design in most cases. Before 1987, only two elbow arthroplasty were performed on patients suffering from severe osteoarthritis as a result of trauma, and the only method available to us was the fully constrained Allopro endoprosthesis.

Between 1987 and 1993 we operated on 31 patients using the Souter-Strathclyde elbow replacement. Twenty-four of them suffered from rheumatoid arthritis, three had primary osteoarthritis, and four had secondary osteoarthritis as a results of trauma.

Very major post-traumatic instability was treated using a custom-made implant made by the Czech company Prospon in one case.

In all our patients who underwent total elbow replacement, we registered one aseptic loosening (constrained prosthesis), two dislocations, and one deep infection treated by removing the implant (Souter-Strahclyde elbow). The operated elbow in the patient with the custom-made Prospon endoprosthesis sometimes gives way in certain positions.

As a brief summary we must underline the fact that the results in cases where the Souter-Strathclyde endoprosthesis is indicated are generally excellent. The complications mentioned have appeared only in patients with severe previous anatomic changes.

We would like to present all the patients who had complications and to try to explain the causes.

Patient 1

The first case involves a 55-year-old woman 3 years after fracture of the lower end of the humerus. After unsuccessful attempts at osteosynthesis, it was necessary to remove devitalized bone fragments of the distal humerus and the patient was referred to us for further treatment (Fig. 1a,b).

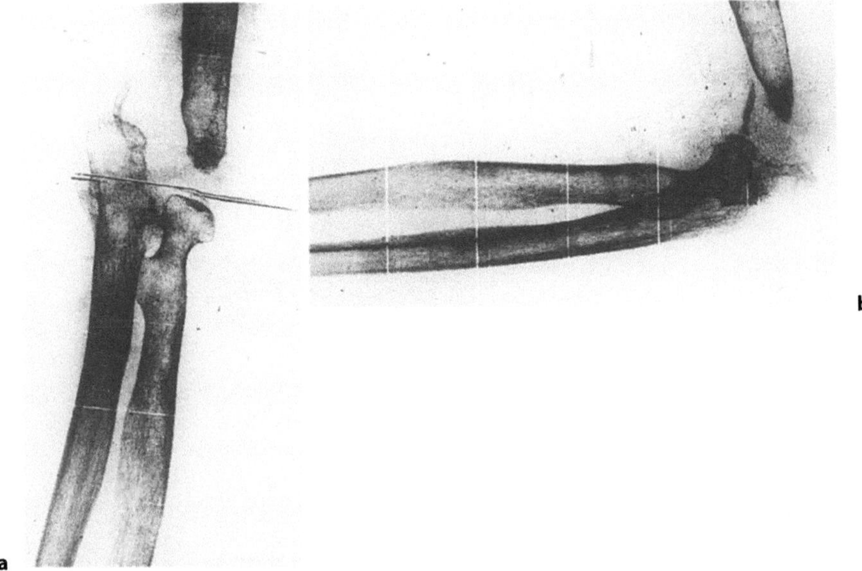

Fig. 1a,b. Patient 1: fractured lower end of the humerus. Devitalized bone fragments of the distal humerus have been removed

Because of a very severe instability of the elbow, we suggested arthrodesis to the patient, but she would not accept it. Therefore, we tried to resolve the situation by using a constrained endoprosthesis (GSB I). Initially, the patient was satisfied. However, she did not follow our instructions and performed heavy manual work. Eight months after the operation, signs of loosening appeared and progressed quite quickly. Two years after the operation major bone defects were evident (Fig. 2a,b). At first, the patient refused reoperation, but her problems finally forced her to agree to it. We took out the loosened endoprosthesis and reimplanted an endoprosthesis with a prolonged shaft on the humeral component. Now, 4 years after reimplantation, the patient is fully satisfied with the results, despite minor signs of loosening.

Patient 2

Another patient was sent to us with very severe post-traumatic instability of the left elbow after an open fracture of the distal end of the humerus with enormous bone loss. Due to major instability of the elbow, a custom-made endoprosthesis was necessary. The implant was made by the Czech company Prospon and its components were similar to the Souter elbow, but joined by a constrained snap-fit system. The distal end of the humeral component was arranged for reinsertion of the muscles of the radial and ulnar humeral epicondyles, but during the operation we found that these muscle groups were attered to such an extent that it was very

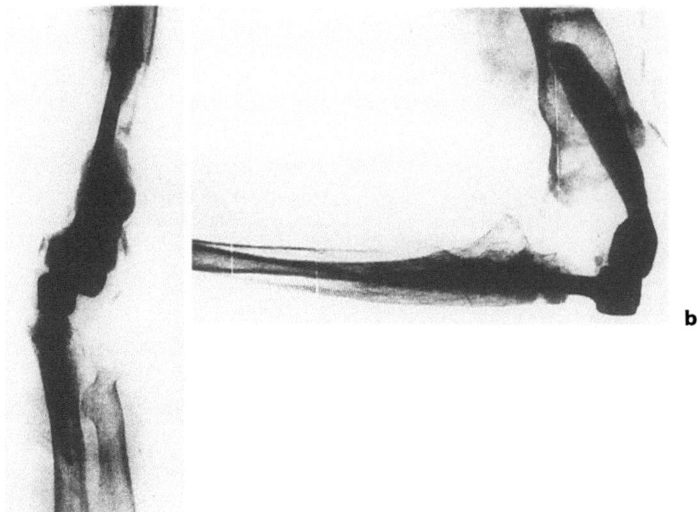

Fig. 2a,b. Patient 1: major bone defects evident 2 years after operation (GSB I prosthesis)

difficult to identify and reconstruct them. We put the operated elbow into a plaster cast for 3 weeks. Then we started careful rehabilitation. In the beginning, stability was good. However, 3 months later symptoms of subluxability appeared. Dislocations followed, but only in pronation (Fig. 3a,b). Two and a half years after the operation the patient is satisfied with the operation, despite subluxations of the elbow, we are considering the possibility of resolving the situation using a constrained type of endoprosthesis. However, the patient is from Slovakia and therefore administrative problems have arisen.

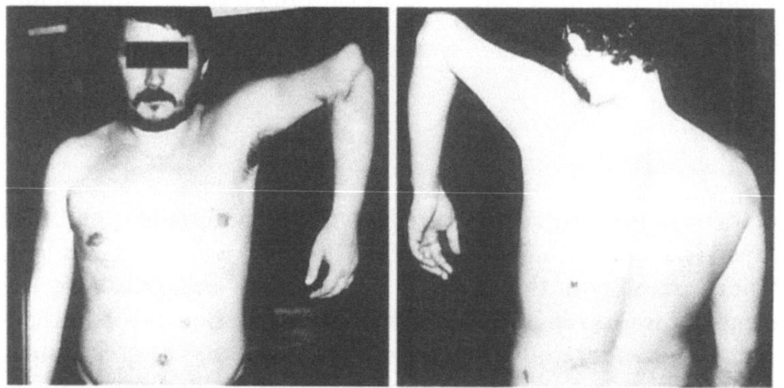

Fig. 3a,b. Patient 2: dislocation in pronation

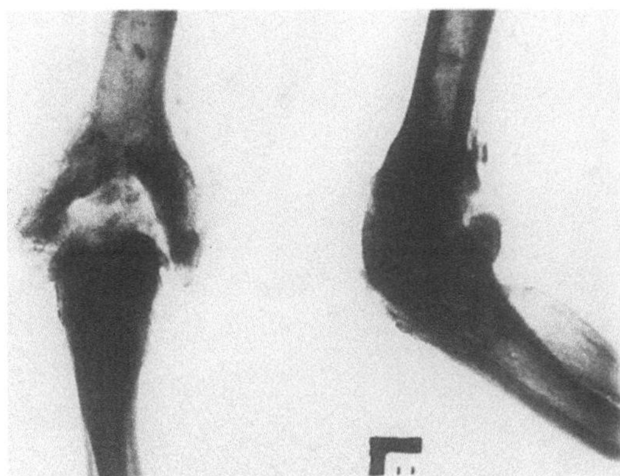

Fig. 4. Patient 3: limited range of motion, though good stability and little pain

Patient 3

The other patient treated elsewhere for an open fracture of the distal humerus and olecranon with several operations, complicated with infection, was sent to our clinic. His elbow was practically ankylosed in an unfavorable position. We implanted a Souter elbow replacement 2 years after the last operation. The implantation was very difficult because of the great amount of para-articular ossifications. Within 3 weeks a wound infection occurred. After one unsuccessful attempt to cure the infection by debridement and irrigation drainage, the endoprosthesis was removed during the second revision due to loosening. The range of motion is currently limited. Fortunately, there is only a little pain and quite good stability of the joint (Fig. 4).

Patient 4

The final patient with complications was a woman who had suffered inveterate traumatic dislocation of the elbow (Fig. 5a). In spite of carefully performed rehabilitation of the operated elbow, a dislocation occurred on the third day. Attempts at closed reduction were unsuccessful, and so we carried out open reposition. The elbow was fixed with a plaster cast; nevertheless, we were not able to maintain the correct position (Fig. 5b). The cause was probably the imbalance of the stabilizers of the affected joint and also the behaviour of the patient, who was mentally ill. We have found a solution for the above-mentioned problem by using external fixation. We used a fixator which enables movement of the elbow joint (Fig. 5c,d), and therefore also functional treatment. External stabilization was applied for 6 weeks. During this time, without the fixater the patient has a range of motion of 30°–120°. She is without pain and is fully satisfied.

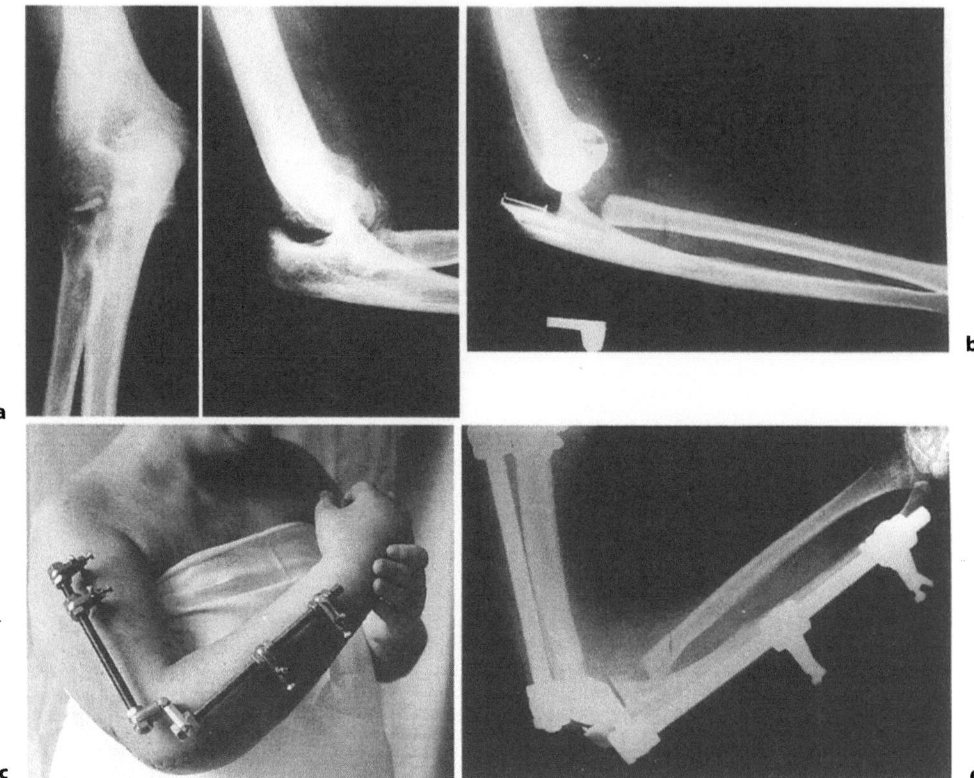

Fig. 5a–d. Patient 4: **a** Traumatic dislocation of the elbow. **b** Correct position cannot be maintained. **c,d** Fixator enabling movement of the elbow

Conclusion

As shown by our complicated cases, it is necessary to decide carefully whether it is possible to perform arthroplasty in cases of great instability of the elbow. The situation is especially problematic in cases of previous dislocations of the elbow. Here, a hinge prosthesis should probably be used.

The Guildford Elbow

P.J. Stiles

The Guildford elbow is a dual-component, unlinked replacement of the humero-ulnar joint and is combined with radial head excision. The prototype prosthesis was developed in co-operation with the Biological Engineering Department of Surrey University, Guildford. The first joint was inserted in 1980. Since then, certain modifications in design and surgical technique have been made as a result of clinical experience. There are right and left components, but only one size of each component [1].

The humeral component (Figs. 1, 2) is cast in chrome-cobalt alloy. Its shape and dimensions were determined by measurement of normal radio-graphs and dry bones. The articular surfaces of the trochlear follow the curves of the normal joint, but the lateral wall of the notch is elongated to produce a symmetrical notch to increase lateral stability.

As a result of the high rate of loosening of hinge prostheses, the fashion had swung to condylar replacement without intramedullary stems. It was, however, felt that the muscular forces acting on the front of the condyles in the functional position of flexion and the necessity to use the arms to assist weight-bearing in many poly-arthritic patients made stem fixation vital for long-term survival. The prosthesis was therefore designed with a 6-cm intramedullary stem, which was offset laterally and posteriorly to the articular portion to reproduce the normal relationship between the axis of the joint and the long axis of the shaft of the humerus.

The intramedullary stem is inserted through the posterior cortex in the supracondylar region and the flattened expanded lower end of the stem fits firmly into the expanded medullary cavity of this region, giving good fixation against rotational forces. The resection of the condylar bone to accommodate the articular portion is minimal and is aligned with the long axis of the humerus by use of a template fitting on the posterior cortex of the shaft. Fixation is by cement.

The ulnar component (Figs. 1, 2) is manufactured in high-density polyethylene. The articular surfaces match those of the trochlear and the intramedullary stem follows the curves of the normal ulna. The carrying angle is reproduced in extension by a 5° angulation of the articular portion of both components to their long axes. The stability of the prosthesis depends entirely on the soft tissues, which must therefore be preserved by a surgical exposure, leaving the medial ligament intact and restoring a normal capsular and ligamentous tension after closure. The correct positioning of the components will then correct any

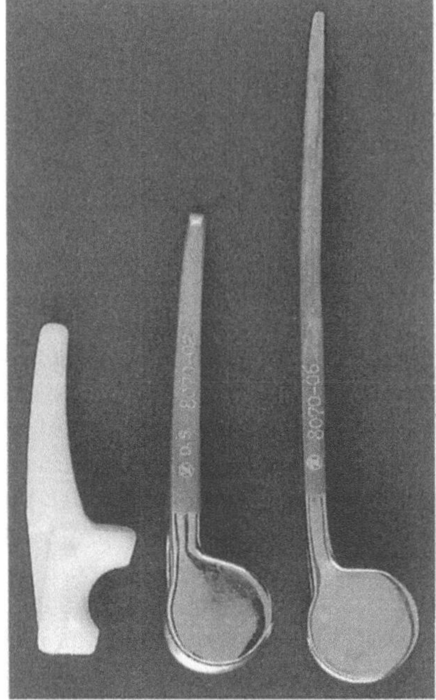

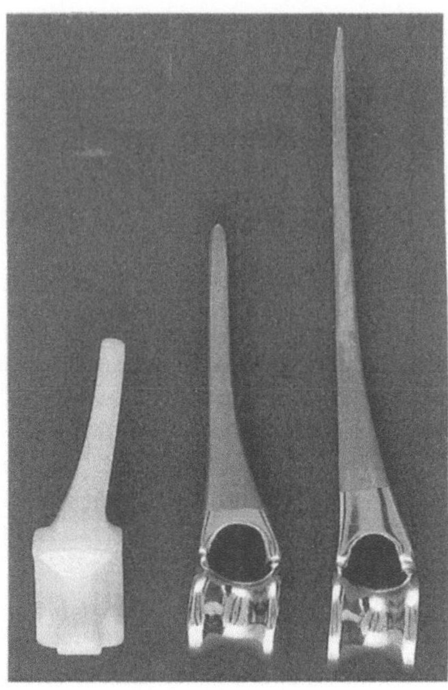

Fig. 1. Lateral views of ulnar component and humeral components with 6-cm and 10-cm stems

Fig. 2. Antero-posterior views of ulnar component and humeral components with 6-cm and 10-cm stems

ligamentous laxity resulting from the bone erosion that frequently occurs in rheumatoid arthritis.

The triceps is split longitudinally, both its aponeurosis and muscle fibres, to its attachment on the lateral side of the tip of the olecranon. The incision is then extended distally along the lateral border of the olecranon to a point immediately distal to the superior radio-ulnar joint. A periosteal flap is then raised from the tip of the olecranon so that the medial portion of the triceps can be retracted medially in continuity with the triceps aponeurosis. It is thought that this minimal disturbance of the triceps mechanism may account for the improved range of extension obtained in 60% of our patients.

A review of the first 49 cases [2] confirmed that the early results were excellent when judged by relief of pain, range of movement, functional improvement and patient satisfaction. The rate of aseptic loosening of the humeral component was, however, unacceptable at 16% with a maximum follow-up of 6 years, the loosening in all of these cases occurring during the first 2 years after insertion. The causes of this were considered under two headings: surgical technique and prosthetic design.

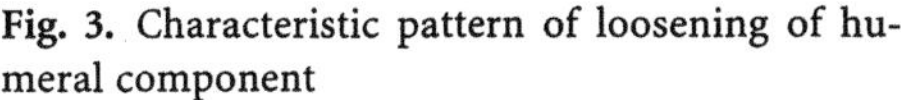

Fig. 3. Characteristic pattern of loosening of humeral component

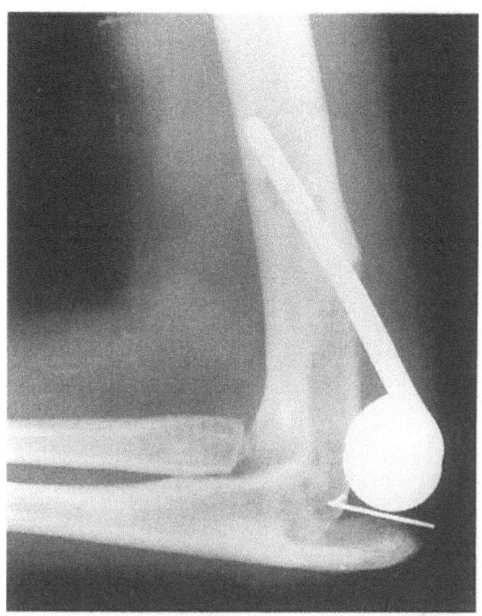

The findings at revision in six patients showed poor cement filling, and the cement technique was improved in subsequent cases using pressure injection by syringe and an intramedullary bone block in suitable cases. A special curette to clear the medullary cavity was also designed.

The pattern of loosening was identical in all cases (Fig. 3), with backward displacement of the articular surface and forward tilting of the stem to expand or erode the anterior cortex. This is due to the strong forces acting on the anterior surface of the condyles mentioned above.

Two modified designs were produced, one with condylar fixation by a lateral and medial expansion (Fig. 4) and a second by increasing the stem length to 10 cm (Fig. 1).

The next follow-up study of the first 80 implants included 23 of these modified prostheses: seven of these were revisions of loosened 6-mm stems to 10-mm stem components without condylar fixation, and the remaining 16 had condylar fixation with variable stem lengths. The length of follow-up of these cases varied between 1 to 7 years, and during this period none of these had developed aseptic loosening. Although the period of follow-up was short, these findings were encouraging because previous loosening had occurred within the first 2 years and five of the revisions to long stems had a period of follow-up exceeding 5 years.

Insertion of the long-stemmed prosthesis is technically easier than the prosthesis with condylar fixation, particularly in rheumatoid patients with extensive bone erosion of the lower end of the humerus. In view of the encouraging results with the long-stemmed model, we are currently using this design only and during the last 3 years have experienced no problems with early loosening. A detailed assessment of our overal results will be ready for publication at the end of this year.

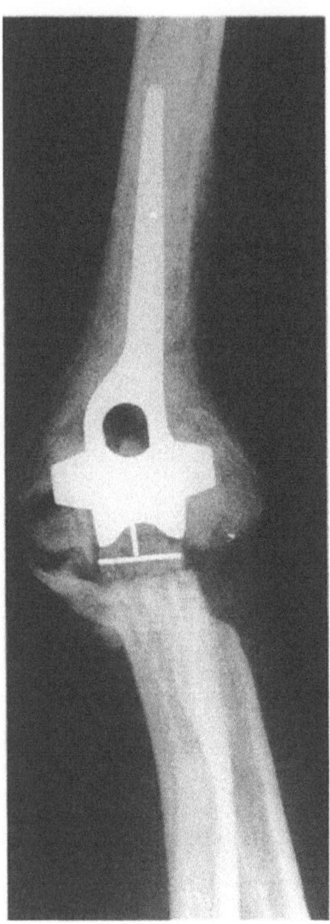

Fig. 4. Humeral component with condylar flanges

Intra-operative fracture has occurred in only three of the first 100 cases, one fracture involving the olecranon and two minimally displaced vertical cracks in the vulnerable medial humeral condyle. These all occurred in small-boned patients and a smaller size of both components may be required to avoid this complication.

Ulnar neuritis has proved a troublesome complication in 12% of patients, marring an otherwise successful operation. Fortunately, this was only serious in 4% of cases, usually being a partial lesion, with rapid recovery. In two patients where the nerve was not transposed, a severe neuritis, with increasing pain, necessitated re-exploration within 6 weeks of operation. In both patients the nerve was involved in dense fibrous adhesions immediately below the medial epicondyle and was adherent to the olecranon process. Following decompression, mobilisation and anterior subcutaneous transposition, the pain was relieved and nerve function slowly recovered.

Our observations lead us to believe that mobilisation of the nerve should be minimal. It should be decompressed within its groove behind the medial epicondyle but left in situ. Auterior transposition should only be performed if the nerve appears to be under tension when the elbow is flexed at the conclusion of the operation.

References

1. Evans EJ, Stiles PJ (1980) The Guildford elbow joint. J Biomed Eng 2:205–210
2. Stiles PJ, Karanjia NB (1990) The Guildford elbow. Int Orthop 14:315–319

Complications and Salvage Procedures

Reconstruction with the GSB III Prosthesis

B.R. Simmen and N. Gschwend

Introduction

Elbow arthroplasty should provide pain relief, restore function, provide normal or close to normal range of motion, and be *salvagable* in case of failure. Therefore, the design of the prosthesis should incorporate the following: (a) minimal bone resection, (b) retaining of the collateral ligaments, (c) possibility of reconstruction of humeral epicondyles, (d) short intramedullary stems (no interference with shoulder arthroplasty in the same arm), (e) provide good clinical long-term results, and (f) design based on sound biomechanical principles to prevent aseptic loosening in the long term.

The main indication for elbow arthroplasty has been rheumatoid arthritis in its late stages (Larsen-Dahle-Eek stages, IV and V). Up to stage Larsen IV bony architecture of the elbow joint is still preserved, even when joint surfaces are completely destroyed. For these cases elbow replacement with a resurfacing prosthesis of the condylar type is possible. However, when the process of destruction has continued beyond stage IV, reconstruction with a prosthesis of the nonlinked type is no longer suitable. Once bony architecture of the elbow joint is completely destroyed, reconstruction is possible only with a linked type of implant.

Post-traumatic osteoarthritis is the second important indication for elbow arthroplasty. Typically these patients have sustained several reconstructive procedures prior to arthroplasty. In most cases bony architecture of the joint is considerably altered, and in many cases one is dealing with condylar or supracondylar nonunion. Reconstruction of these cases by arthroplasty is technically demanding. The prosthesis must provide options to reconstruct bony architecture, restore physiological biomechanics (joint axis), and reconstruction of soft tissues, namely extensor apparatus and collateral ligaments. In the presence of bone loss and loss of soft tissues this can be difficult.

All elbow prostheses which have been implanted in greater numbers are designed for cement fixation of at least the humeral component. This includes also the GSB III prosthesis. Aseptic loosening normally means considerable bone loss in the area of the epicondyles and significant thinning of the cortical bone within the range of the cement cone. The anatomy of the distal humerus with the shape of the medullary canal changing from a circular form to a very flat ellipsoid form further distally practically precludes the stable insertion of a stem without additional fixation by bone cement. This situation is entirely different, however, in the case of aseptic loosening, suggesting other solutions for fixation of the prosthesis in case of revision.

Design Principles of the GSB III Prosthesis

The GSB III prosthesis is a linked elbow joint. Mechanically it is a sloppy hinge. The stem of the ulnar component can glide in the high-density polyethylene bushing of the humeral component. Axial deviation between ulnar and humeral component is possible within a range of 8° with respect to varus and valgus as well as flexion and extension. Rotation of the ulnar component relative to the humeral component is possible within a similar range. Both components have a stem, introduced into the medullary canal of humerus and ulna. The articulation of the prosthesis allows reconstruction, of the physiologic center of rotation of the elbow joint. In addition to the intramedullary stem, fixation of the humeral component is achieved by *anterior* and *distal flanges* which support both humeral condyles anteriorly and distally. Implantation of both components requires little bone resection and allows retention of both collateral ligaments [3].

Since its introduction in 1978 the GSB III prosthesis has been used without modification for 16 years [1, 3]. Recently a larger joint in addition to the previously available sizes has been added. Improved instrumentation facilitates accurate implantation and is designed similarly to the new instrumentations for knee arthroplasty.

Designed for cement fixation, the prosthesis is made of a cromium-cobalt alloy (Protasul 10 und Protasul 2). For severe revision cases a custom-made titanium humeral component for fixation without cement has been introduced. Because of the conical shape of the humeral intramedullary stem this component is not suitable for primary implantation (Fig. 6).

For implantation of the GSB III prosthesis the presence of *humeral condyles* is compulsary. Forces from lower arm to upper arm are introduced into the distal humerus via the *flanges* of the humeral component and into the humeral epicondyles. This fact is of crucial importance in the presence of severe bone loss by rheumatoid arthritis, posttraumatic bone loss, or bone loss because of a failed implant.

It has been shown by Gschwend [2] that reconstruction of missing or destroyed condyles is possible by using autologous bone graft from the iliac crest (Figs. 1, 2). In addition, the flanges of the prosthesis facilitate reconstruction of the condyles with bone grafts at the time of primary arthroplasty and revision (Fig. 1).

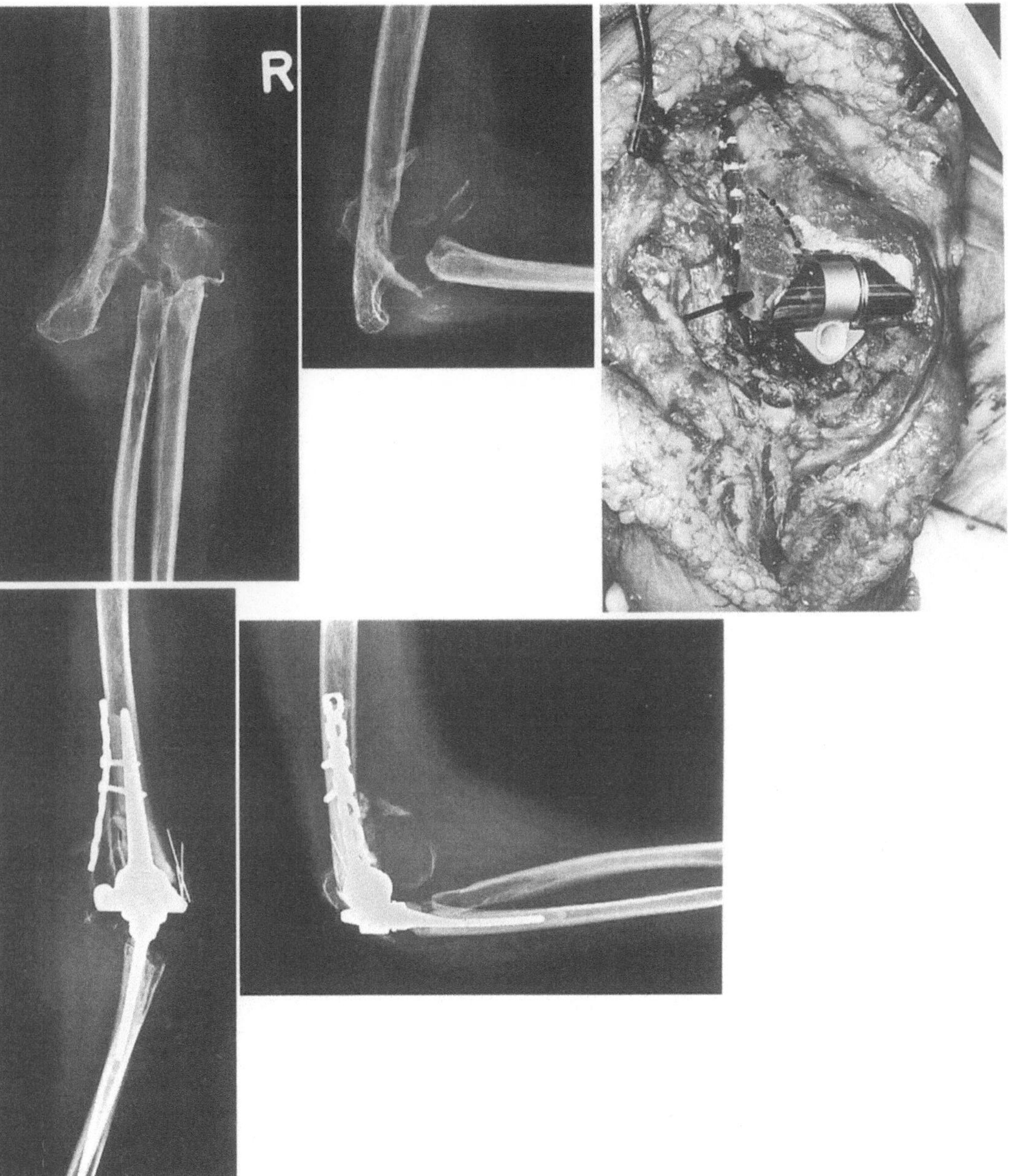

Fig. 1a–c. "Flail" elbow of a 46-year-old woman with long-standing mutational rheumatoid arthritis. **a** Severe bone resorbtion with pathologic fractures of ulnar epicondyle and olecranon. Total elbow arthroplasty with GSB III prosthesis incorporating reconstruction of the ulnar epicondyle with autologous bone graft from the iliac crest (internal fixation with AO 3.5-mm DC plate) and augmentation of radial epicondyle with bone graft (fixation with K wires). **b** Intraoperative situs. **c** Result 2 months postoperatively

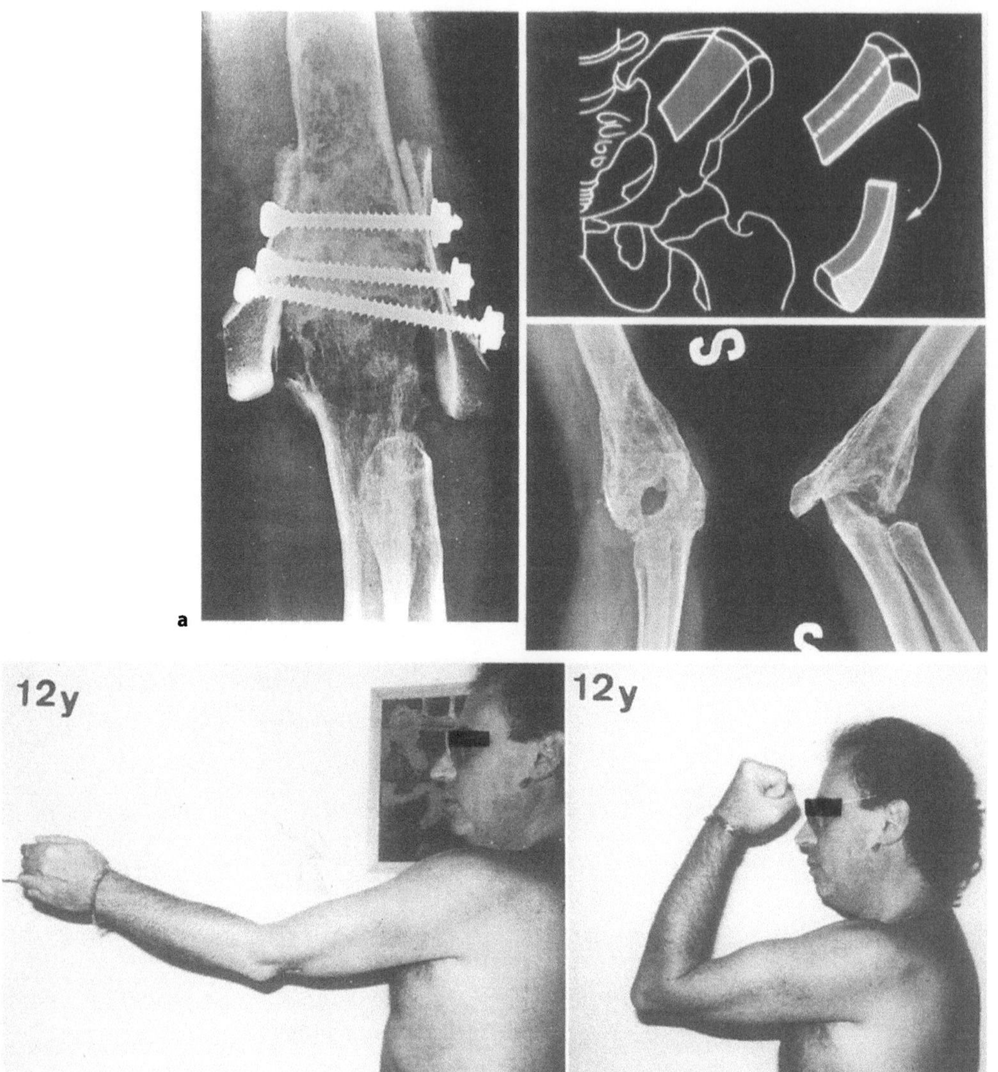

Fig. 2a–d. Reconstruction of humeral epicondyles after removal of loose failed DEE prosthesis with autologous bone grafts from iliac crest as described by Gschwend. **a** Postoperative X-ray. **b** Schematic description of procedure. **c** Radiological result 6 years postoperatively. **d** Functional result 12 years after removal of failed DEE prosthesis and conversion to resection arthroplasty with reconstruction of humeral condyles. Because of acceptable pain relief and function patient did not wish reimplantation of a new prosthesis

Reconstruction of the Flail Elbow in Rheumatoid Arthritis

Long-standing RA can lead to severe destruction of the elbow joint. Normally a V-shaped, forklike distal humerus is preserved which articulates with a very thin olecranon. These severely involved joints often cause very little pain. However,

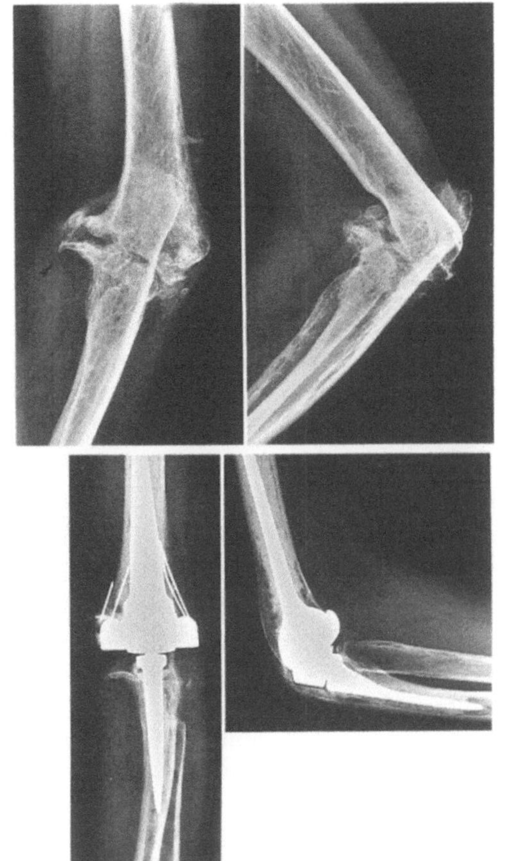

Fig. 3a,b. Left elbow of 49-year-old woman with long-standing rheumatoid arthritis. **a** Twelve years after resection arthroplasty. **b** Two years after GSB III elbow arthroplasty with augmentation of both humeral epicondyles with autologous bone grafts fixed with K wires

they are unstable and interfere with practically all activities of daily life. The situation is further complicated by fracture of one or both condyles or the olecranon (Fig. 1). Creation of a stable, mobile, and pain-free joint with elbow arthroplasty is possible. Using the GSB III prosthesis, reconstruction of the humeral epicondyles is mandatory. If there is no local bone graft available (radial head) incorporation of an autologous bone graft from the iliac crest is recommended (Fig. 1). Similar conditions can be expected after synovectomy and radial head excision as primary treatment of rheumatoid elbow involvement. Depending on the long-term therapeutic effect of synovectomy concerning pain relief, function, and stability, arthroplasty can become a necessity. In most cases there is enough bone stock left for solid fixation of the humeral component. Bone from osteophytes and/or the intercondylar resection can be used for reconstruction of the epicondyles. In our experience fixation with K wires has been sufficient (Fig. 3). To achieve union after reconstruction of a spontaneously fractured olecranon does not seem possible. In two cases we have left it in place, functioning similarly to a patella, to protect the triceps tendon from the prosthesis.

Posttraumatic Osteoarthritis and Supracondylar Nonunion

The majority of our patients with posttraumatic osteoarthritis who have needed elbow arthroplasty had been operated on once or several times before. Intra-articular fractures of the distal humerus are difficult to treat; nonunions have a poor prognosis. Even when bony fusion can be attained, the joint will probably remain painful. Total elbow arthroplasty can be a successful treatment option in such cases (Fig. 4). Spontaneous fusion of the elbow enlarges the lever arms at the fracture site. It may prevent healing and lead to nonunion. In such an elbow motion occurs in the nonunion and very probably is severely reduced and painful. Arthroplasty may be the only predictable treatment option (Fig. 5).

Failed Prosthesis

Infection

In the series from 1978 to 1992 there were 3/118 deep infections in rheumatoid arthritis (2.5%). Among the posttraumatic cases one of 26 elbows became infected. All four elbows had to be revised and were converted to resection arthroplasties after removal of the implants and all bone cement. Since both humeral epicondyles were preserved, in all three cases acceptable range of motion and stability with little pain was achieved. Reimplantation of a total elbow would theoretically be possible; however, the patients were satisfied with the final result and did not wish such a procedure.

For late infections three therapeutic possibilities have been discussed in the literature. In addition to, removal of the prosthesis and convertion to a sine-sine type of arthroplasty, arthrodesis and reimplantation of a new elbow prosthesis are possible. In the case of a first-time infection by gram-positive bacteria, we would today consider replacing the infected elbow implant simultaneously by a new prosthesis in a one-step operation. However, in the case of recurrent infection, gram-negative bacteria, and/or extensive damage of bone, a two-step operation with reimplantation of a new prosthesis after an interval of 6–8 weeks is a safer procedure with better prognosis for healing of the infection. In our opinion, arthrodesis must be considered only exceptionally.

Aseptic Loosening

The GSB III elbow design has been very successful concerning aseptic loosening in long-term follow-up. Among the series of 144 elbow arthroplasties performed from 1978 to 1992 there was no complete radiologic loosening in the rheumatoid

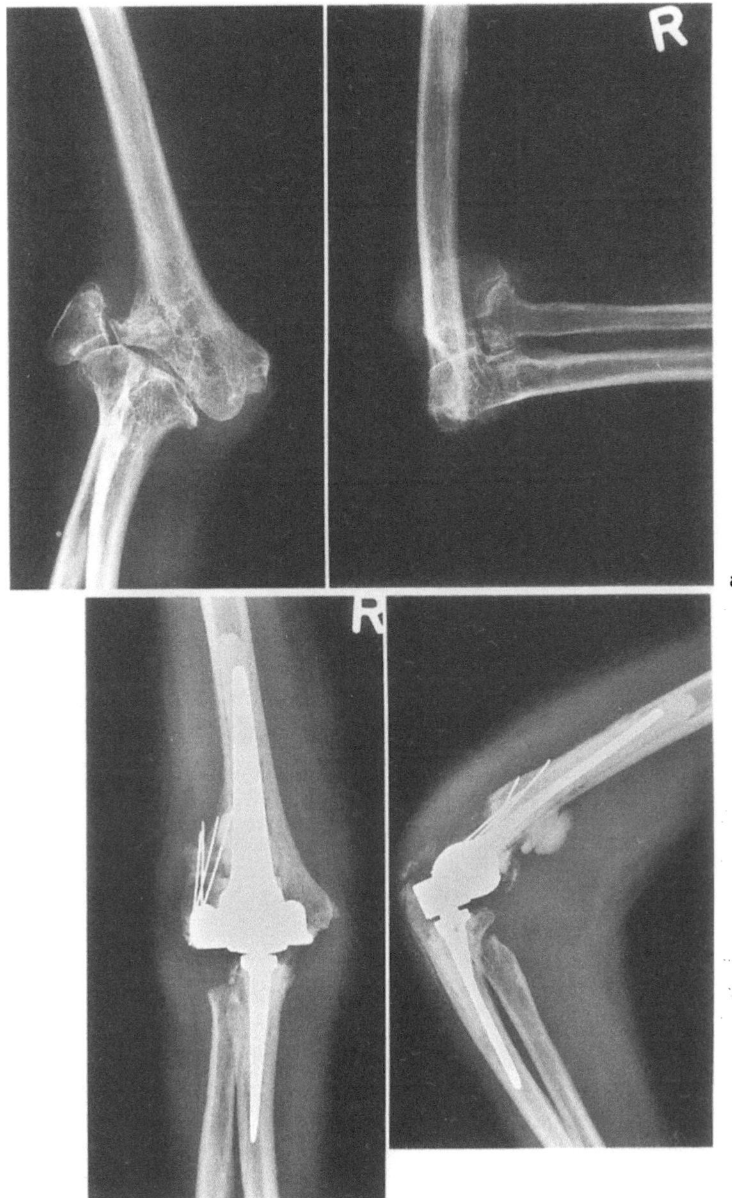

Fig, 4a,b. Painful posttraumatic osteoarthritis of the right elbow of 50-year-old woman with nonunion of radial epicondyle. **a** Severe loss of function and instability after several attempts of reconstruction. **b** Total elbow arthroplasty using a GSB III prosthesis incorporating reconstruction of radial epicondyle. By incorporating the capitellum into the reconstruction collateral ligaments were stabilized at the same time

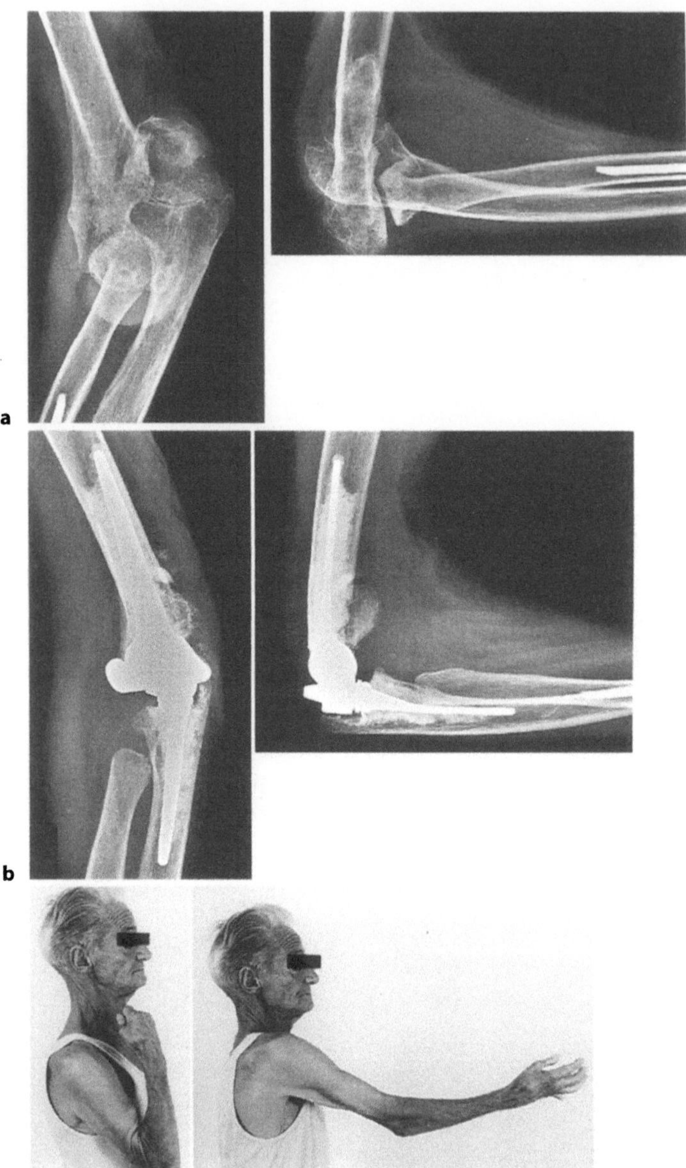

Fig. 5a–c. A 76-year-old patient with long-standing rheumatoid arthritis. **a** X-ray of right elbow 14 years after supracondylar fracture which led to nonunion and bony ancylosis of the humero-ulnar joint. Because of increasingly painful stiffness and instability the patient wished treatment by arthroplasty. On the opposite elbow he had an arthroplasty 12 years earlier with flawless function. **b** GSB III arthroplasty was performed. Because of precarious soft tissue situation it was not possible to restore anatomical length. To prevent uncoupling of the prosthesis the ulna lengthening device was used. **c** Excellent range of motion after reconstruction

arthritis cases ($n = 118$) and only one case of loosening with migration in a 35-year-old manual worker 3 years after arthroplasty in the posttraumatic osteoarthritis group ($n = 26$; Fig. 6). Since 1992 bilateral loosening of both components in a rheumatoid arthritis patient 5 years postoperative was noted. Radiologic loosening of the humeral component with scalopping probably due to high-density polyethylene wear, without migration of the implant, was found in an other rheumatoid patient. However, this patient is free of symptoms and is not yet ready for revision.

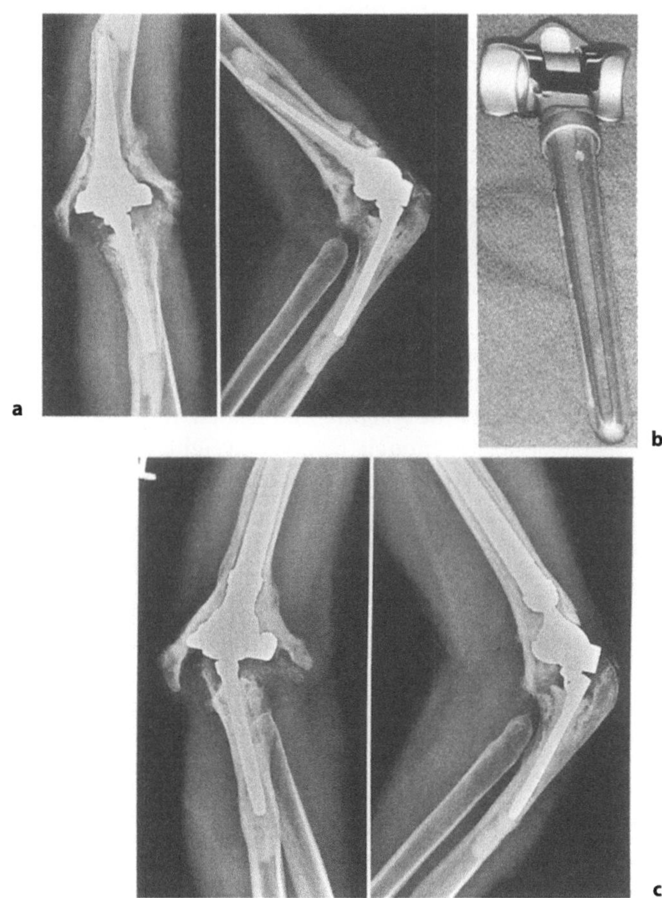

Fig. 6a–c. First case of aseptic loosening of a GSB III elbow prosthesis 3 years after implantation in an 38-year-old manual laborer with posttraumatic osteoarthritis. **a** Preoperative X-ray demonstrating radiologic loosening, migration of the prosthesis, and fracture of the humerus. **b** The implant and all bone cement were removed, and reconstruction with a custom made prosthesis (humeral component) with conical titanium stem for cementless implantation was performed. **c** Three years after reimplantation the fracture was healed, and considerable new bone formation around the titanium stem was noted. The patient is pain free, has good range of motion of his stable elbow joint, and is able to work

Our experience with revision of failed elbow arthroplasties is derived from the early GSB I implants (before 1978) and from revision of other than the GSB prostheses. The GSB I prosthesis was a hinged metal to metal elbow of the first generation which led to loosening of the humeral components in 30% of the cases during the first 5 years. However, in contrast to other designs, the GSB I prosthesis needed very little bone resection. Revision of these cases was therefore quite straightforward. The humeral epicondyles were still intact and bone stock allowed the insertion of a new cemented GSB III prosthesis. The length of the intramedullary stem of the two implants is practically equal.

Loosening of the humeral component in an active young manual worker 3 years after GSB III arthroplasty to treat severe posttraumatic osteoarthritis has led us to a different approach for this problem. Encouraged by the success of similar designs for revision of failed hip arthroplasties, we replaced the loose humeral component after removal of all bone cement with a custom-made humeral prosthesis with a conical intramedullary titanium stem designed for cementless fixation. The shaft was long enough to secure fixation proximal to the fractured diaphysis (proximal tip of the former implant). The midterm result (3 years) is very promising. The diaphysial fracture healed rapidly within months, and 3 years after revision considerable new bone formation is visible leading to solid incorporation of the new prosthesis (Fig. 6). The same concept has since been used successfully for revision of a loose Coonrad prosthesis with severe bone loss and multiple pathologic fractures of the humerus. Three months postoperatively the fracture had healed, new bone formation was visible, and the arm was stable enough to allow weight bearing. In a third case the custom-made titanium humeral component was used to treat a periprosthetic fracture. In an elderly rheumatoid patient a GSB I elbow prosthesis was implanted in 1976. After 14 years revision was necessary because of aseptic loosening. The GSB I prosthesis was replaced by a cemented GSB III prosthesis. Four years later the 82-year-old patient sustained a periprosthetic fracture of the humerus by a trauma. Instead of performing an internal fixation the stable GSB III prosthesis and all bone cement were removed, and a custom-made titanium humeral component was introduced which stabilized the fracture at the same time. Healing occurred within 3 months, allowing pain-free and stable elbow function. This type of design may in the future prove useful as primary arthroplasty of choice in particular cases.

According to most other authors, the therapy of loosening consists of reimplantation of a prosthesis with a longer stem and, where necessary, of bone grafts. Arthrodesis should be regarded as a very last resort. Convertion into a sine-sine type of arthroplasty is usually also unsatisfactory.

If the humeral condyles were resected at the time of implantation of the first prosthesis, or if these are partly or totally resorbed, we recommend reconstruction of the epicondyles with bone grafts from the iliac crest [2] (Fig. 2). The technique was originally described to improve resection arthroplasty; today we would advise simultaneous implantation of a GSB III prosthesis after reconstruction of the condyles (Fig. 1).

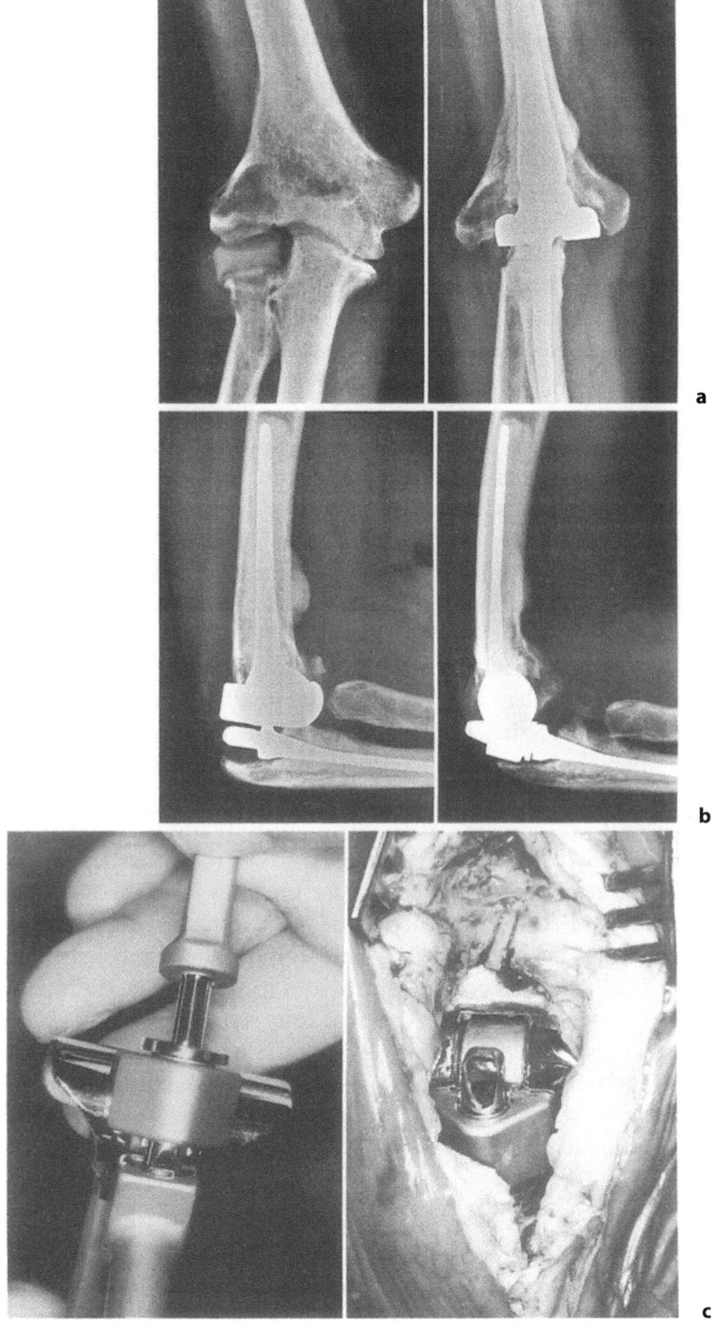

Fig. 7a–c. A 42-year-old woman with posttraumatic osteoarthritis of the right elbow. **a** Prior to arthroplasty radial head replacement with a silicone prosthesis was performed (**a**), which lead to bone resorbtion in the opposite capitellum. Because of increasing pain and stiffness GSB III elbow arthroplasty was performed 10 years ago. Ten years postoperatively uncoupling of the prosthesis occurred (visible in lateral view), which made revison necessary. **b** After recoupling of the prosthesis incorporating the ulna lengthening device the patient remained free of pain. **c** Ulna lengthening device (*left*) before and after implantation (*right*)

Uncoupling: A GSB III Prosthesis Related Complication

Spontaneous disassembly or uncoupling of the "articulation" of the prosthesis was the main complication encountered in the early days of 16 years experience with the GSB III prosthesis. Uncoupling occurred in 5 cases of 118 rheumatoid arthritis elbows (4.2%) and in 4 of 26 posttraumatic cases (15.3%). Two main factors lead to disassembling: 1) too extensive soft tissue release, and/or 2) incorrect location of the center of rotation; the instant point of the sloppy hinge not corresponding to that of the anatomical elbow, being generally too proximal.

Reconstruction of normal anatomy with an elbow prosthesis is difficult to achieve in posttraumatic cases where normal anatomy is altered, and more extensive soft tissue release is necessary to achieve sufficient mobility of previously stiff joints. Since we have learned to position the center of rotation more precisely, "uncoupling" has become a rare event. The new instrumentation has also contributed to a more accurate positioning of the implants. In addition, this complication can be prevented in high-risk cases by using a supplementary element which lengthens the ulnar component of the joint. This lengthening device is used routinely when revising disassembled prostheses (Fig. 7).

In *summary*, total elbow arthroplasty with the GSB III elbow prosthesis provides good or excellent long-term results in a high percentage of the cases. The design principles of this implant restore normal biomechanics, preserve bone stock, namely the humeral epicondyles, and preserve soft tissue stability (collateral ligaments). The rate of aseptic loosening in the first 10 years is very low, and the overall success rate over 90%. The preservation of the humeral epicondyles facilitates revision when necessary. On the other hands, reconstruction of the humeral epicondyles is crucial for the long-term success with this type of implant. A method for reconstruction of the condyles with autologous bone grafts (iliac crest) has been presented. The combination of reconstruction of bone stock and GSB III elbow arthroplasty provides the experienced elbow surgeon with a tool to salvage even desperate cases of long-standing rheumatoid arthritis with severe bone loss and cases of posttraumatic osteoarthritis with destruction of normal elbow architecture, including nonunion of the distal humerus. A new concept for revision of failed implants with severe bone loss and/or fracture of the humerus is described.

References

1. Bell S, Gschwend N, Steiger U (1986) Arthroplasty of the elbow. Experience with the mark-III-GSB prosthesis. Aust NZ J Surg 56:823
2. Gschwend N (1983) Salvage procedure in failed elbow prosthesis. Arch Orthop Surg 101:95–99
3. Gschwend N, Löhr J, Ivosevic-Radovanovic D, Scheier H, Munzinger U (1982) Semi constrained elbow prostheses with special reference to the GSB III prosthesis. Clin Orthop 232:104–111

Revision Total Elbow Replacement

M.P. Figgie

Introduction

Advances in surgical technique and implant design combined with the recognition of the importance of restoring the anatomic relationships of the elbow have led to a decreased complication rate associated with total elbow arthroplasty. However, when failure do occur it may lead to a very complex situation. The surgical solutions for the failed total elbow replacement are usually extremely challenging with high complication rates. The options range from implant removal with resection arthroplasty to revision total elbow arthroplasty to even amputation in severe cases. When faced with a failed total elbow replacement, the surgeon must understand the failure mode, evaluate the remaining soft tissues, bone, and neurovascular status, and then individualize the treatment option for the patient.

Failure Modes

The most common types of failure necessitating revision elbow replacement include: (a) loosening, (b) infection, (c) instability, and (d) prosthetic failure involving either polyethylene wear or implant fracture. Periprosthetic fractures which require revision may also occur but are usually associated with loosening. Other causes for poor results include nerve dysfunction, triceps insufficiency, and stiffness; however, these usually do not require revision of the prosthesis.

Loosening

Aseptic loosening is usually felt to be an implant-specific complication, with nonconstrained implants having lower loosening rates than semiconstrained and constrained devices. Theoretically, nonconstrained implants rely on soft tissue stability secondary to ligament support. Thus, loosening rates should be lower because stresses are absorbed by the ligaments and are not transferred directly to the bone–cement interface. However, these prostheses are usually utilized in patients with rheumatoid arthritis and marked osteopenia secondary to steroid use, and loosening can occur. Still, most authors have noted low revision rates for humeral loosening with the capitellocondylar prosthesis, with rates ranging between 0% and 2% [5–7, 29, 31, 34, 39]. The rates of ulnar component loosening have been higher, but the revision rates have been similar [5–7, 29, 31, 34, 39]. Other nonconstrained-type devices have had higher rates, especially those without humeral stems. The rates of revision for loosening have ranged up to 36% [15–17, 24, 25, 30, 32, 33, 35, 38]. In addition, Kudo documented a 70% humeral subsidence rate with humeral components without stems [15].

Semiconstrained implants have been associated with higher rates of revision for loosening, ranging between 0% and 14% [1, 2, 4, 9, 13, 14, 19, 22, 23, 26, 28, 37] (Fig. 1). The early Coonrad and Mayo devices had revision rates reported at 14% and were later modified to provide more laxity at the articulation [4, 22]. With this modification, there have been no revisions for loosening in the latest study with follow-up ranging from 2 to 8 years [19]. In addition, Figgie and associates reported no revisions for loosening among 137 semiconstrained implants using both the triaxial and Osteonics devices at up to 13-year follow-up [9].

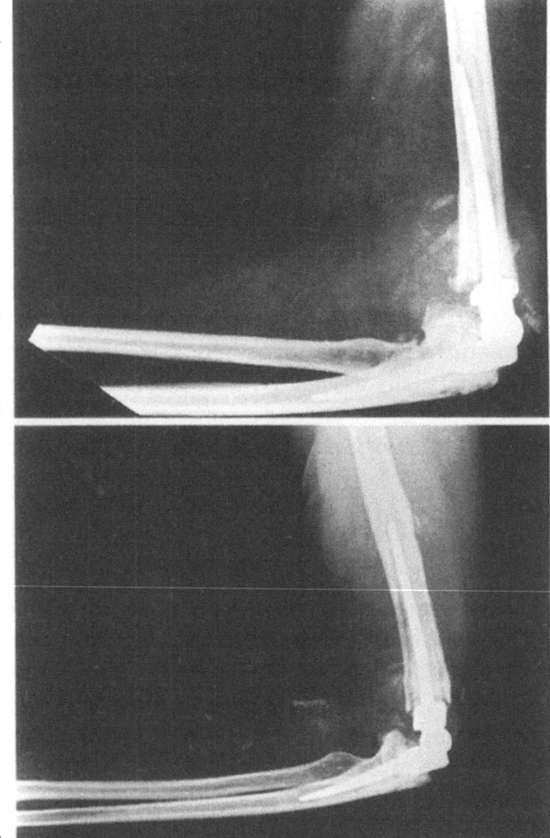

Fig. 1. a This patient with post-traumatic arthritis had revision, which went on to have humeral loosening with typical posterior migration with anterior migration of the tip. **b** This was revised to a longer-stemmed prosthesis

The fully constrained devices such as the Dee and Gschwend-Scheier-Bähler (GSB) provided excellent initial results, but had high failure rates as a result of loosening [11]. This was due to the high stresses at bone–cement interface caused by implant constraint combined with particulate debris from the metal-on-metal articulation. In addition, several of the designs required complete resection of the distal humerus, including the origins of flexor and extensor muscles. The loss of the soft tissue supporting sleeve created further stress on the bone–cement interface and resulted in failure due to rotational stresses and torsional loads.

Septic Failure

Deep infection is one of the most devastating complications of total elbow replacement (Fig. 2). The rates of infection have ranged from 0% to 11%, but in the larger

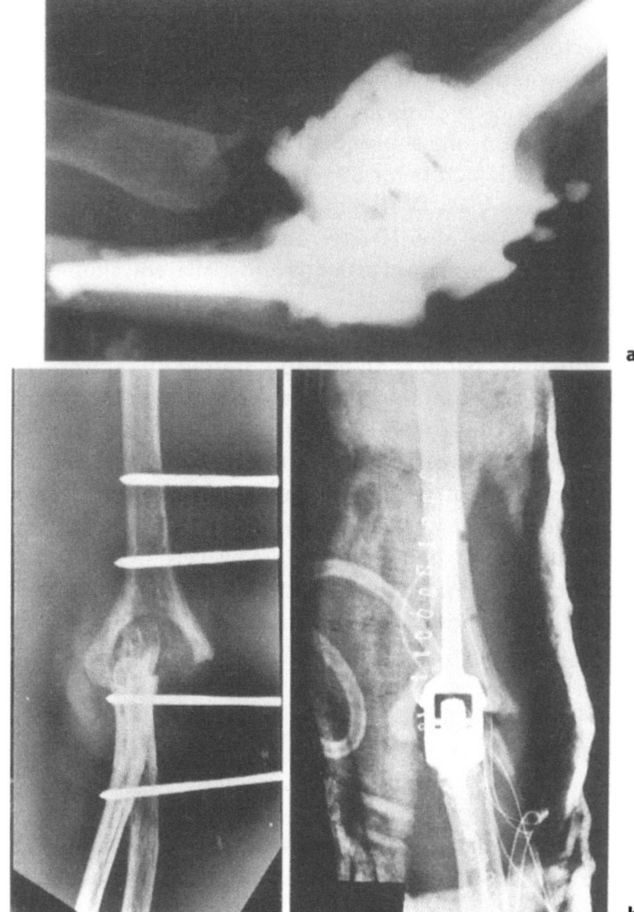

Fig. 2. a An infected total elbow after an arterial catheterization which became infected. The arthrogram shows a small sinus pocket. **b** The elbow was removed, cement was debrided, and the patient's arm was placed in an external fixator. **c** After 6 weeks of antibiotic treatment, the elbow was successfully reimplanted

series Morrey and Bryan reported a 9% infection rate [20] and Wolfe and associates reported a rate of 7.3% [40]. However, the risk of infection has decreased due to improvements in surgical technique and the use of antibiotic-impregnated cement in some series. Kraay and associates reported no deep infections in primary total elbow replacements for rheumatoid arthritis since the introduction of antibiotic-impregnated cement in 1986 [14]. In spite of these improvements, however, the risk of infection still exists due to several reasons. First, the lack of subcutaneous tissue about the elbow makes it more vulnerable to pressure and skin necrosis. In addition, total elbow replacements are usually performed on patients with severe rheumatoid arthritis or post traumatic arthritis. The patients with end-stage rheumatoid arthritis are often on disease-modifying antirheumatic drugs, including methotrexate as well as corticosteroids. These patients also place a great deal of pressure on the elblow as they often use them as weight-bearing joints during ambulation on platform crutches. Patients with post-traumatic arthritis have often had previous operations compromising skin vascularity and increasing the risk of wound healing.

In the series by Morrey and Bryan and by Wolfe and associates, several risk factors for infection were evaluated [20, 40]. Patients undergoing primary total elbow replacement have a higher risk for infection if they have had any previous elbow surgery. This increase was 12% in Morrey's study and 19% in Wolfe's study. In addition, any subsequent surgery placed the elbow at a risk of infection of 20%. Other risk factors for infection included previous infection of the elbow, psychiatric illness, class IV rheumatoid arthritis, postoperative wound drainage, spontaneous drainage after 10 days, and ipsilateral shoulder arthritis [40]. The patients with class IV rheumatoid arthritis and ipsilateral shoulder arthritis tend to place greater demands upon the elbow. Morrey and Bryan showed significantly increased risk for infection with steroid use, while Wolfe and colleagues had a 7% risk of infection with those patients undergoing steroid therapy as opposed to 6.6% of those not on steroids. Combining the two series, the responsible bacteria was *Staphylococcus aureus* in 18 elbows, *Staphylococcus epidermidis* in five, and a different organism in each of five remaining elbows. Nine of these infections occurred between 3 months and 1 year, while ten occurred after 1 year. The clinical presentation of these patients was extremely varied. In Wolfe's series, 12 of 14 patients had severe pain and 12 had drainage. However, only seven had increased temperature, whereas five had erythema and four had swelling. Radiolucency was detected in ten of the 14 elbows, but only four had the scalloping that is typical of infected joint replacements.

Instability

Nonconstrained Prostheses. Instability may occur in nonconstrained implants if soft tissue balance is not present (Fig. 3). Instability may range from subluxation or translocation to frank dislocation. Usually those patients with translocation where the ulnar component articulates with the capitellum are functioning well and do

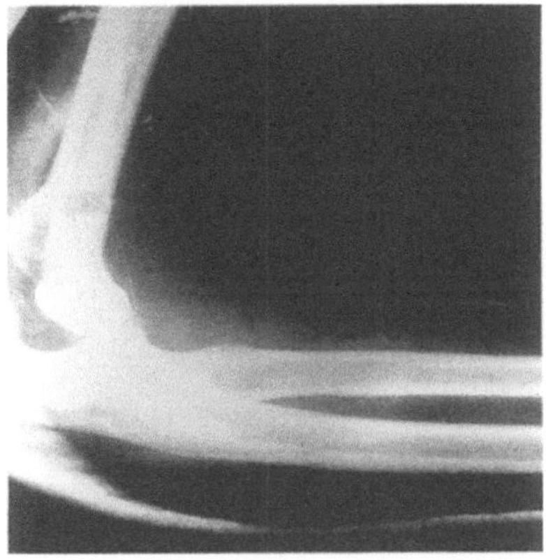

Fig. 3. An unstable capitellocondylar replacement. Options for treatment include casting, revision of the humeral component, exploration of the medial side, or revision to a semiconstrained device

not require revision surgery. Frank dislocation has occurred in 3%–15% in series of capitellocondylar implants [5–7, 29, 31, 34, 39]. In the majority of these series, the dislocations were initially treated by closed reduction and casting for a 4-week period, after which the elbows were gradually mobilized. This form of treatment was successful in more than 50% of the reported cases. In other cases, the medial side of the elbow was explored, and attempts were made to reconstruct the medial collateral ligament. The results of this procedure have been inconsistent [5–7, 15, 16]. Other options for unstable nonconstrained implants include revision of the humeral component to increase the carrying angle, which tightens the medial soft tissue tension. This has been described in one case each by Ewald and colleagues, Tuke, and Rydholm [7, 30, 35]; it was successful in two of the three reported cases. A final option for patients with recurrent instability is revision to a semiconstrained implant.

Semiconstrained Prostheses. Instability among semiconstrained prostheses has been rare, except with the Pritchard-Walker and triaxial components. The other semiconstrained devices are usually linked, and dislocation only occurs when the locking mechanism has failed. In a study on the original Pritchard-Walker implant, ten out of 269 cases had instability due to faulty locking of the axial pin [23]. Instability in the triaxial implant is secondary to polyethylene failure (Fig. 4). Figgie and associates reported eight late dislocations [26] after 4 years. This led to the redesign of the triaxial implant to change the load-bearing surface from the condyles to the central region to improve stress distribution and decrease polyethylene wear. In addition, a non-load-bearing restraining axle was added to prevent dislocation.

Implant Fracture

Nonconstrained Prostheses. There have only been two reported fractures in nonconstrained prostheses, both of which were capitellocondylar devices with

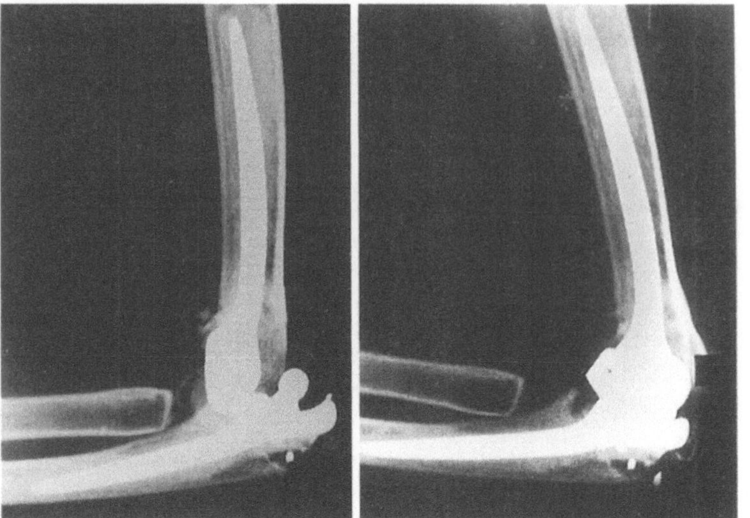

Fig. 4a,b. This triaxial component dislocated 4½ years after implantation secondary to polyethylene wear. The bushing was revised and an anterior yoke was added

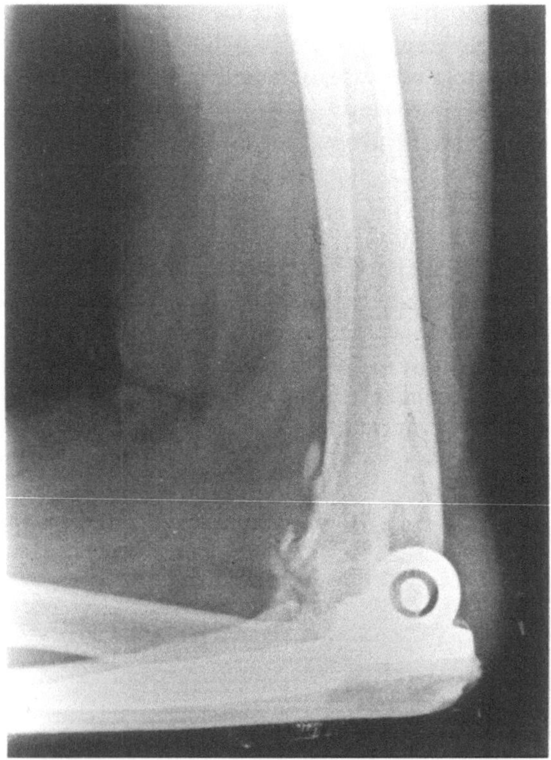

Fig. 5. This Pritchard-Walker implant fractured. The all-polyethylene humeral component fractured, requiring revision to a type-2 humeral component

all-polyethylene ulnar components. One fracture, reported by Rosenberg and Turner, occurred 36 months after surgery as a result of a traumatic incident [27]. The second fracture, reported by Ruth and Wilde, was noted on a 12-year follow-up radiograph [29]. Neither of the patients with fractured prostheses has undergone revision surgery.

Semiconstrained Prostheses. The original Pritchard-Walker implant had a high failure rate due to fracture of its all-polyethylene humeral component (Fig. 5). Pritchard reported eight humeral component fractures among 269 implants for a rate of 3% [23].

There has been only one reported fracture of a metal total elbow component; this was reported by Morrey and Adams, who had a patient fracture the ulnar component of a Coonrad elbow replacement 27 months after surgery [19]. This patient had resumed heavy labor, which may have contributed to the fracture. The patient did require revision of the ulnar component.

Initial Evaluation

Evaluation of the failed total elbow replacement may be extremely complex. As reported by Wolfe et al. [40], the initial presentation of an infected elbow replacement may be varied. Thus, any patient who presents with a painful elbow should be evaluated for a possible infection. The same is true for any patient who presents with a loose total elbow replacement. In evaluating the failed total elbow replacement, a careful physical examination must be performed. Blood tests are often not helpful, as patients with rheumatoid arthritis often have elevated sedimentation rates. However, a high white cell count with a shift may be suggestive of infection. With regard to physical examination, evaluation of the patient's motion is appropriate, especially if there has been any change in that motion over the recent time period. The elbow should be evaluated for stability and swelling. In addition, evaluation of nerve function is critical, especially the ulnar nerve. However, radial and median nerves should not be ignored. Skin incisions must be carefully evaluated, and the patient's biceps and triceps power must be determined.

High-quality X-rays are important in evaluating the failed total elbow replacement. These are important to evaluate the radiolucencies, and comparison to previous X-rays are important. Loosening may present with minimal changes, but in other instances there can be gross bone destruction due to particulate debris. Cortical thinning may occur with "ballooning" of the humerus or ulna. Bone resorption can also occur. In a frequent pattern of loosening, the distal humerus will migrate posteriorly with the tip migrating anteriorly. The bone should be evaluated for possible fractures, especially at the level of the epicondyles. If there is any question as to the bone stock remaining, then computed tomography (CT) scans are helpful in determining bone geometry. In the loose total elbow replacement or the possible infected elbow replacement, aspiration should be performed. Bone scans may be helpful in the work-up of a potentially infected elbow, but we find no use for magnetic resonance imaging (MRI) in a failed total elbow replacement. An electromyograph (EMG) is often an excellent preoperative study in patients who present with any neurologic dysfunction.

In cases where there may be elbow instability that is not demonstrable on plain X-rays, fluoroscopy is useful. This can evaluate potential subluxations in patients with nonconstrained implants.

Treatment Options

Treatment options for the failed total elbow depend upon the mechanism of failure. With the septic elbow, options include the following:

1. Debridement with antibiotic suppression
2. Implant removal with arthodesis
3. Implant removal with resection-type arthroplasty
4. Two-stage reimplantation

With a loose total elbow, options include implant removal with:

1. Arthrodesis
2. Resection-type arthroplasty
3. Revision surgery

With the unstable total elbow replacement, operative treatments include the following:

1. Reconstruction of the medial collateral ligament
2. Addition of a thicker polyethylene component
3. A change in the valgus angle of the humeral component
4. Revision to a semiconstrained implant

With the unstable semiconstrained implant, revision of the polyethylene with or without the addition of yoke can be considered. However, revision to a linked component may be required if the components are malaligned. With a fractured component, revision of that component is required.

Arthrodesis

Arthrodesis of the elbow is an operation to be avoided whenever possible. Loss of motion at the elbow is extremely disabling, and patients find that they are unable to perform most activities of daily living. Arthrodesis is only considered for the failed total elbow if there is loss of the humeral epicondyles such that the elbow would be flail (Fig. 6). In this instance an arthrodesis would be deemed preferable to a flail elbow or an amputation. Arthrodesis after a failed elbow replacement, however, is extremely difficult to achieve due to marked bone loss.

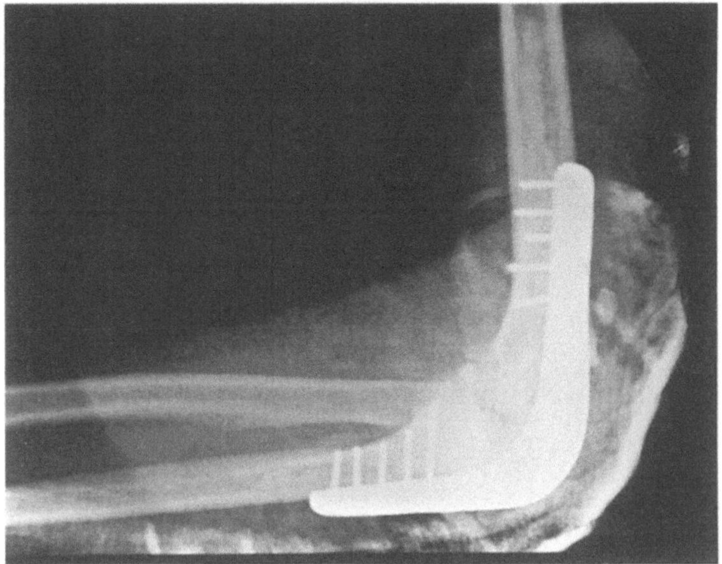

Fig. 6. Arthrodesis after a failed total elbow replacement is difficult to achieve due to a loss of bone stock. Function is diminished due to the loss of motion. However, this may be the only option for a flail elbow

Resection Arthroplasty

Preferred treatment for an infected total elbow replacement where reimplantation is not considered is a resection-type arthroplasty. This is a modified resection, as the original resection arthroplasty first described by Verneuil in 1860 [36] included removing the distal humerus above the epicondyles along with resection of a portion of the olecranon and excision of the radial head. This leaves the elbow as a flail, useless joint. Currently, with an infected elbow we will remove the implant and all cement and place the patient in an external hinged device. This provides for soft tissue healing while maintaining stability of the elbow. The goal is to achieve an anatomic reduction of the olecranon within the humeral epicondyles (Fig. 7). The hinged device will allow for early range of motion and provide alignment of soft tissues and healing in the plane of motion [10]. The fixator is usually used for a 6- to 8-week period and the pins are placed under direct vision to prevent injury to the radial nerve on the lateral side and the ulnar nerve on the medial side. In a series of patients undergoing removal of failed total elbow replacements, Figgie and associates reported that seven of eight patients who achieved an anatomic alignment had satisfactory results [10]. All eight elbows were pain free with an average arc of motion of 85°. Flexion was usually excellent, but triceps strength was often compromised. No excellent results were obtained, but there was only one failure secondary to a radial nerve palsy. Among the three patients in whom an anatomic reduction could not be achieved, all experienced failure and two required arthrodesis.

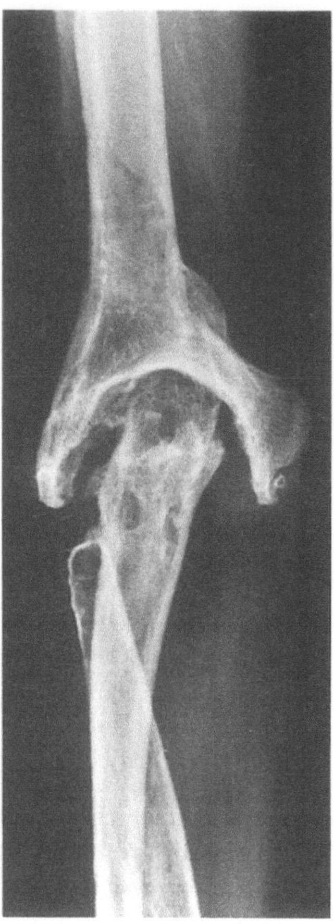

Fig. 7. Patients with failed total elbow replacements may do well with a resection-type arthroplasty if an anatomic reconstruction can be obtained with containment of the olecranon within the epicondyle

Antibiotic Suppression

Antibiotic suppression alone is not recommended. It should be combined with debridement and a 6-week course of i.v. antibiotics followed by oral antibiotic suppression. This should only be considered for sensitive bacteria and well-fixed components. There is an extremely high failure rate: in the series by Morrey and Bryan, only one of 14 elbows was salvaged by suppression, and in Wolfe and associates' series only three of 13 elbows were successfully treated by suppression [20, 40].

Reimplantation

Reimplantation after infection is performed rarely and only in carefully selected patients. Primary selection criteria include the ability to eradicate the infection adequately as determined by minimum inhibitory concentration levels and the presence of adequate bone stock with sufficient soft tissues. We recommend the removal of the original infected elbow replacement and all the cement and the replacement of an external fixator for 3–4 weeks. This should then be removed and the patient placed in a removable splint while i.v. antibiotics are continued. The proper antibiotic levels must be obtained according to the minimum inhibitory concentration levels. Reimplantation can be considered after 6 weeks of antibiotic treatment. In general, reimplantation is recommended only when resection arthroplasty has failed as a result of pain or instability.

Surgery For Instability

Nonconstrained total elbow replacements that are unstable (in the early perioperative period) and have had a frank dislocation are usually treated by a 4-week period of cast immobilization. However, for patients who fail that treatment or have late dislocations, then one option is exploration of the medial elbow with reefing of the capsule, reconstruction of the medial collateral ligament, and post operative immobilization. However, the results are unpredictable, especially in patients with rheumatoid arthritis where soft tissues may be marginal.

Humeral Component Revision

Another option that exists for the unstable nonconstrained elbow is to revise the humeral component to one that has an increased valgus angulation. This will tighten the medial structures and may improve the instability. However, one must be aware of the increased angulation of the humerus, which changes the carrying angle and kinematics of the elbow. Motion may be altered if significant changes occur. In addition, the ulnar nerve may be subject to tension, which might result in an ulnar neuropathy. The other option is to place a new ulnar component with a thicker component, which would serve to tighten the joint and the existing soft tissues. However, if this fails, then revision to a semiconstrained implant would be the procedure of choice.

Polyethylene Revision

In the unstable semiconstrained devices, the source of instability must be identified. If there is failure of the locking mechanism this may be able to be revised, although sometimes the locking mechanism has been deformed and the humeral component would require revision. With the triaxial component, failure occurs secondary to polyethylene wear and revision of the polyethylene bushing provides stability. In many instances, a yoke is also applied in order to provide increased compression and reduce instability. However, this technique was successful in only 50% of the cases as reported by Gerwin and associates [12]. In patients with malposition of their components, according to the criteria of Figgie et al. [8], revision of polyethylene bushing alone will most likely not provide satisfactory results and revision of the components will be required.

Revision Surgery

Implant revision is the procedure of choice in patients with loose components who have adequate bone stock for reconstruction. Patients with fractured components may also successfully undergo revision of the fractured component.

Preoperative Planning For Revision Surgery

In addition to thorough clinical evaluation and X-ray evaluation, there are several factors that must be considered prior to revision surgery. Soft tissues must be adequately evaluated including muscle strength. Neurologic evaluation is also critical, as is bone quality. In patients with questionable bone defects, a CT scan is often helpful in order to evaluate this further.

The revision implant is critical in the procedure. Often a standard type of device may be utilized for revision if the bone structure is maintained. However, in those cases where there is loss of humeral bone, a long-stemmed version may be required. In cases where there is loss of one or both epicondyles, we recommend the use of an anterior flanged device to help decrease rotational stress. Customized devices may be required to maintain the center of rotation. With standard long-stemmed devices, the canal will determine the center of rotation. In addition, humeral canal diameters vary markedly and components may need to be altered to fit. Longer-stemmed devices are recommended when there are perforations or fractures, and these devices should bypass defects by two bone diameters. However, one must be aware of interference with the humeral stems of shoulder re-placements, especially in patients with multiple joint arthritis. Usually ulnar components only need to vary based upon stem length and diameter. In cases where one is revising only the humeral component of a nonconstrained device, the appropriate humeral components must be available at different valgus angulations.

In addition to having the proper implant available, one must also be prepared for nonprosthetic options, including an external fixator as a temporizing measure if revision cannot be performed.

If significant bone loss is present on preoperative evaluation, one should be prepared for bone grafting. This may involve either preparation of the iliac crest or access to bone bank graft. In complex cases where soft tissue coverage may be difficult, preparation for skin grafts or muscle flaps may be necessary. This may involve a preoperative evaluation by a plastic surgeon or surgeons specializing in soft tissue coverage.

With regard to special instrumentation, several tools are helpful in removing cement and prostheses. A full array of instruments for removing the implant should be available, especially with linked snap-fit link devices, where special tools may be required for disassociating the component. Cement removal instruments, including the small-tip and small-bore Midas (Midas Rex, Ft. Worth, TX, USA) can be helpful. In addition, ultrasound devices with small attachments are extremely helpful in removing cement from the shaft of the ulna and humerus. Fiberoptic lights of small diameter are also useful in evaluating the canal.

Implant Selection

In general, we find that nonconstrained components are difficult to utilize as revision prostheses. They are dependent upon soft tissue support and after failure of a prosthesis the ligamentous stability is suspect. Thus, in almost all instances, revision surgery should be done with a semiconstrained-type component. The decision to use a standard or customized component is based upon available bone quality. As previously mentioned, if there is a bony defect, a long-stemmed device should be utilized. However, too long a stem should be avoided, as it can interfere with the humeral component of a shoulder replacement by creating a large stress riser and may alter the accurate positioning of the center of rotation, as stem length and size will determine where the center of rotation is placed. In addition, anterior flanges may be useful to help with rotational stresses, but again may force the center of rotation into a particular position if the flange ends up determining the rotation of component (Fig. 8). Customized implants may be required in order to accurately place the center of rotation within the available bone stock. However, there is a learning curve associated with custom components with regard to design, proper fit, and implantation. The use of cementless components for revision surgery is still considered experimental.

Surgical Technique

The usual surgical approach that we employ for revision operations is the Bryan-Morrey posteromedial reflection of the triceps [3]. However, in many instances the implant can be disarticulated without reflecting the triceps, thus preserving the triceps attachment. The approach should be made through a previous skin incision, if at all possible; however, if the approach was on the lateral side and a posteromedial approach is being used, then a new incision should be made in order to avoid large flaps. If there is any question about the skin incision, preoperative evaluation with a plastic surgeon may be indicated.

With the posteromedial approach, the patient is placed in a supine position and the arm is brought up in a position over the chest. The skin incision is made over the medial border of the triceps and extended to the level of the cubital tunnel. The incision then curves to the proximal third of the ulna. Subcutaneous tissues

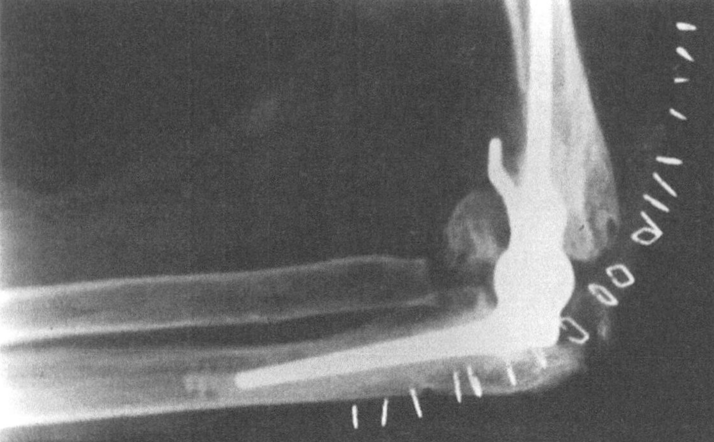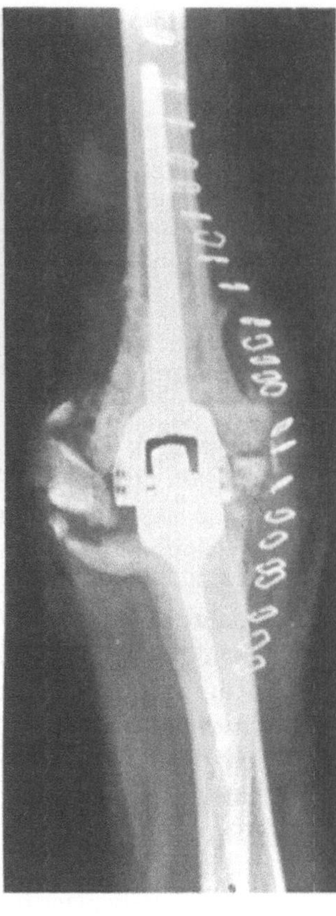

Fig. 8a,b. Patients with loss of the distal humerus may require an anterior flange to help with rotational control. Note the suture holes (**b**) within the component for attachment and stabilization of the soft tissue sleeves

are divided and subcutaneous flaps are avoided. The ulnar nerve is identified at the cubital tunnel and is dissected free along its course proximally and distally. With revision surgery, the surgeon must be aware if the ulnar nerve was transposed with the original operation. This should be reviewed from the old operative notes. When the nerve has been operated on previously and there is scar tissue, the proximal incision may need to be extended and the nerve found at the medial border of the triceps and carefully followed distally. The ulnar nerve must be identified, free, and protected in any revision operation. A Penrose drain (Sherwood Medical, North Brunswick, NJ, USA) is placed around the nerve and sutured instead of using a clamp in order to avoid undue tension. The nerve is dissected free and a passage is created between the two heads of the ulnar flexor muscle of the wrist to allow the nerve to be translocated anteriorly. The fascia of the ulnar flexor muscle of the wrist is then divided to the proximal third of the ulna, from where the ulnar nerve enters underneath the fascia. The triceps muscle is dissected free medially and elevated laterally, with care taken to avoid injuring the ulnar nerve that lies within the fibers of the proximal triceps muscle. If an extensile exposure is required, then the triceps attachment is elevated at the tip of the olecranon along with the periosteum. A Beaver blade (Becton-Dickinson, Mountain View, CA, USA) is helpful in performing this. The sleeve of the triceps and the forearm fascia remain in continuity and are elevated across the capitellum to the lateral epicondyle, exposing the radial head. The anconeus muscle is also reflected. The capsule and scar tissue are excised and the medial aspect of the olecranon is exposed. The ulnar flexor muscle of the wrist is reflected to the sublime tubercle and the medial collateral ligament is subperiosteally elevated. The ulnar nerve is carefully protected as it lies in close proximity to the sublime tubercle. At this point the locking mechanism of the component can be removed and the elbow can be dislocated.

Another way to approach a revision is to perform the posteromedial incision and dissect the ulnar nerve free. The triceps is then elevated both medially and laterally from the humerus, the locking mechanism of the device is identified, the coupling mechanism is removed, and the humerus and ulna are disassociated. The medial collateral ligament is reflected and the olecranon can be exposed, leaving the triceps mechanism intact. The ulnar nerve must be carefully protected to ensure that no undue tension is placed. Once the ulna and humerus are exposed, then an anterior capsulectomy is performed by placing a hemostat anterior to the capsule and excising it down to the brachial muscle. At this point the original prosthesis can be removed. If it is loose, it may be easy to remove; however, one must be careful if the cement is well fixed to the component, because fractures may occur in trying to remove a large piece of cement. If the implant is well fixed, then the implant can be removed before the cement is addressed. In cases of infection, all cement must be removed, whereas in cases of revision for dislocation or aseptic loosening well-fixed cement does not need to be removed if it does not interfere with the new implant. Removal of cement from the ulna and humerus is extremely difficult due to the small caliber of these bones. Most hand tools are still too large to remove the cement. We avoid utilizing the Midas instruments, except where excellent visualization and control can be obtained. The Midas may chatter enough to cause perforations or fractures of the humerus or ulna, which creates a great deal of difficulty with the revision operation. In addition, perforations of the proximal humerus place the radial nerve at risk. If there is any question, the midshaft of the humerus must be well exposed and, in some cases, the radial nerve identified and protected. If the Midas equipment is to be used, then the small diameter of barrels must be obtained in order to be effective. We currently prefer using the small tips on the ultrasonic devices, which allow for safer cement removal within the shaft. However, even this can cause perforations in soft rheumatoid bone. If there is a great deal of difficulty removing the cement or if there is an inaccessible area, a cortical window or a posterior trough may be required. However, creating a posterior trough in the humerus will reduce the support for the revision prosthesis. The posterior cortex is extremely important, as the vector force from the joint reaction force causes posterior loading. Most humeral components loosen by migrating posteriorly with the tip perforating anteriorly. During cement removal cultures should be taken and frozen sections identified in order to rule out a subclinical infectious process in the case of loose components.

When removing fractured implants, the preparations for removing the distal stem must be made. This may involve the use of a special Midas device to drill the stem and remove it. However, this can be extremely difficult due to the small diameter of the component. A cortical window may be required in order to remove it.

With the ulna, a large subperiosteal reflection might be necessary in order to avoid perforation. Due to the angulation of the shaft of the ulna, cement removal with straight instruments is difficult. The small-tip ultrasonic devices are again extremely helpful and, as in the humerus, well-fixed cement does not need to be removed for noninfectious revision surgery.

Once sufficient cement has been removed, bone defects must be identified. Perforations should be grafted. If defects are significant in important areas, such as the posterior aspect of the humerus, then cortical strut grafts may be utilized along with morselized graft. The stems of the components should bypass any cortical defects by at least two bone diameters. If one or both of the humeral epicondyles has been fractured, these should be fixed to the humerus with pins or screws, if feasible. The screws must be of the same type of metal as the humeral component in order to avoid a "battery" reaction due to dissimilar metals. If the epicondyles are not repairable, we often place large Tevdek sutures (Becton-Dickinson, Mountain View, CA, USA) through then and tie this behind the humeral component in order to preserve the soft tissue sleeve. In some instances we have created a custom implant with attachments on the humeral component to allow repair of the soft tissue sleeve or an epicondyle to the component (Fig. 8).

Once the trial components have been placed, range of motion should be tested. The component must track appropriately and the rotation must be judged. This is sometimes difficult due to the loss of normal structures, but the humeral component should be internally rotated approximately 5° with respect to the epicondyles. One must be assured that the humerus is not lengthened, as this may cause undue stress and loss of motion. It can cause greater problems with the polyethylene bushing due to the increase in the joint reaction force. The center of rotation should be maintained and can be moved slightly proximally, but should not be moved distally in the humerus. Once the components have been tested, the canals can be irrigated and dried. We recommend the use of antibiotic-impregnated cement with all revisions. In addition, we utilize methylene blue in the polymethylmethacrylate in case another revision is required. Often, an intramedullary plug cannot be utilized with long-stem components. The humeral and ulnar components can be cemented with the same batch of cement, but with difficult situations, such as a humeral nonunion or fracture, then the implants should be cemented separately. During the cementing procedure, the perforations are exposed in order to prevent cement extrusion and possible damage to the radial nerve along the distal humerus. Cement is trimmed, the tourniquet released, bone grafts placed, including strut grafts, and hemostasis obtained. The elbow is reduced, the components articulated, and the locking mechanism placed. The wound is closed over drains and the triceps muscle is restored by repairing the fascial sleeve. Sutures placed through drill holes in the olecranon help reinforce the repair. The ulnar nerve is evaluated and transposed with a fascial sling, if necessary. The soft tissues are closed and the elbow is placed in a bulky dressing with a plaster splint which is split posteriorly to avoid pressure on the olecranon.

Postoperative Management

The splint is left in place and the wound is inspected after 3 days. If the wound is intact, then early range of motion can be started. An EZ-form splint (Smith Stephens, Memphis, TN, USA) is made in order to protect the arm and is utilized with straps to alternate extension and flexion when the arm is at rest. The splint is usually discontinued after 6 weeks. A therapist guides the patient through the early rehabilitation stage, but the patient is encouraged to use the arm as much as possible for all activities of daily living except for lifting. Flexion is usually regained more easily than extension, as most activities of daily living require flexion. Pronation and supination are also stressed during rehabilitation.

Revision of Polyethylene Bushing for a Triaxial Component

The surgical approach in revision of polyethylene bushing for a triaxial component is similar, utilizing either a triceps flap elevation or dislocation of the component by elevating the triceps medially and laterally after identifying the ulnar nerve. There is often metal synovitis, which must be thoroughly debrided. The bushing may be fragmented and should be removed in its entirety. Exposure of the distal humerus must include removal of a portion of the epicondyle in order to have adequate access to the distal humerus. In some cases, the small bearings are difficult to remove from the sides of the humerus. The new high-density polyethylene bushing should be tested to ensure it fits appropriately. Two small O-rings should be imbedded in the polyethylene with the chamfer facing inwardly. The polyethylene is then fitted to the humerus and the ulnar component is re-duced. This requires considerable force. The yoke, if it is to be used, can be placed from a posterior position. Formerly, we placed it anteriorly, but since its purpose is to squeeze the polyethylene and not block flexion, we find it works equally well from a posterior position. The small screws are then placed through the yoke and humeral component until they are just inside the edge of the yoke. Range of the motion should be tested to make sure that there is no restriction. If there is, the screws are loosened slightly. Then, a small osteotome is used to score the threads, preventing the screws from backing out. The wound can then be closed in the previously described manner.

Results

The largest series of revision total elbow replacement was reported by Morrey and Bryan, with 33 revisions performed over a 10-year period with an average 5-year follow-up [21]. The cause of failure leading to revision was different for these patients, with pain being a common symptom to all. Loosening of the components was the most common factor leading to revision, as 17 elbows had loose humeral components, three elbows had loose ulnar components, and eight elbows had both components loose. Of these, six elbows had fractures of the humerus or ulna due to bony resorption around the loose prosthesis. Three implants had material failure, and two implants were unstable. Eighty-eight percent of elbows had moderate or severe bone loss, with loss of the trochlea or humeral condyles. Two thirds of the patients had rheumatoid arthritis.

Reimplantation was performed with six different commerical prostheses and four custom prostheses, making a comparison of survival analysis difficult. Half of the implants had a long-stemmed humeral componant. Nine percent of the revision prostheses became infected (three of 33), which is similar to the incidence of 7%–9% found in the literature for primary elbow arthroplasties [20, 40]. No mention was made of whether antibiotic-impregnated cement was used, and perhaps this could account for the lower than expected incidence of infection after revision surgery. Rheumatoid patients faired better after revision elbow surgery, with 64% having a good result compared with 40% of those with traumatic arthritis. Rating was based on a scale previously described by Morrey and Bryan evaluating pain, function, and stability [20]. The success of the reimplantation could be correlated to the adequacy of the cementing technique. Neither the number of prior procedures, nor the amount of bone loss at the time of revision was correlated with subsequent failure of the revision prosthesis. Cementation technique was considered inadequate if the cement did not extend beyond the tip of the prosthesis and there was greater than a 1-mm gap over greater than one half of the cement–prosthesis interface on the postoperative anteroposterior or lateral radiograph. Of those humeral components judged to have adequate cementation on postoperative radiographs, none became loose. Of those humeral components having inadequate cementation, 38% loosened (five of 13). All of the ulnar components were judged to have adequate cementation techniques postoperatively, and 10% loosened. Sixty percent of patients had an intraoperative or postoperative complication. In all, one third of revision prostheses (11 of 33) required a second operation to remove or revise the prosthesis for infection, loosening, implant failure, or instability. Of the eight revised prostheses (second revision), five had a good result.

At recent follow-up, 55% of these elbow replacements are still in place with a satisfactory result [18]. Eleven elbows had an additional procedure performed. Evaluation of 47 revision prostheses implanted over the past 5 years has demonstrated improved survival using an anterior flanged Coonrad III implant [18]. Survival rates for 5 years now are 95%.

Results of revision of semiconstrained triaxial total elbow replacements for failure of the polyethylene articulation and resultant dislocation have been fair

[12]. The mean time from elbow implantation to initial dislocation was 30 months. Fifty percent of elbows required more than one revision for polyethylene failure and dislocation. All elbows that dislocated within the first year after implantation redislocated. Radiographic evaluation revealed all implants were outside the acceptable alignment criteria for good outcome of elbow arthroplasty [8].

Conclusion

Revision total elbow surgery is technically demanding with high complication rates. It requires precise preoperative planning and a surgeon prepared to utilize any of several surgical options during surgery. Satisfactory results can be achieved in complex cases.

References

1. Brumfield RH Jr, Volz RG (1981) Total elbow arthroplasty; a clinical review of 30 cases employing the Mayo and AHSC prostheses. Clin Orthop 158:137
2. Bryan RS (1977) Total replacement of the elbow joint. Arch Surg 112:1092
3. Bryan RS, Morrey BF (1982) Extensive posterior exposure of the elbow: a triceps-sparing approach. Clin Orthop 166:188
4. Coonrad RW (1982) Seven-year follow-up of Coonrad Total elbow replacement. In: Inglis AE (ed) Upper extremity joint replacement. Mosby, St Louis
5. Davis RF, Weiland AJ, Hungerford DS et al (1982) Non-constrained total elbow arthroplasty. Clin Orthop 171:156
6. Dennis DA, Clayton MD, Ferlic DC et al (1990) Capitello-condylar total elbow arthroplasty for rheumatoid arthritis. J Arthroplasty 5[Suppl]:583
7. Ewald FC, Scheinberg RD, Poss R et al (1980) Capitellocondylar total elbow arthoplasty: two-to-five year follow-up in rheumatoid arthritis. J Bone Joing Surg 62A:1259
8. Figgie HE, Inglis AE, Mow CS (1986) A critical analysis of biomechanical factors affecting functional outcome in total elbow arthroplasty. J Arthroplasty 1(3):169–173
9. Figgie MP, Inglis AE, Figgie HE III, Mow CS (1990) Semiconstrained total elbow replacement in rheumatoid arthritis. Orthop Trans 14:104
10. Figgie MP, Inglis AE, Mow CL et al (1990) Results of reconstruction for failed total elbow arthroplasty. Clin Orthop 253:123
11. Garrett JC, Ewald FC, Thomas WH, Sledge CB (1977) Loosening associated with GSB hinge total elbow replacement in patients with rheumatoid arthritis. Clin Orthop 127:170
12. Gerwin M, Figgie MP, Mabery JD, Inglis AE (1993) Results of revision of semiconstrained total elbow replacement for dislocation. Presentation, the 60th annual meeting of the American Academy of Orthopaedic Surgeons, San Franciso
13. Inglis AE, Pellicci PM (1980) Total elbow replacement. J Bone Joint Surg 62A: 1252
14. Kraay MJ, Figgie MP, Inglis AE et al (1992) Survivorship analysis of primary total elbow arthroplasty with a semi-constrained prosthesis. Presented at the American Association of Orthopaedic Surgeons, 59th annual meeting, Washing DC
15. Kudo H, Iwano K (1990) Total elbow arthroplasty with a non-constrained surface replacement prosthesis in patients who have rheumatoid arthritis: a long-term follow-up study. J Bone Joint Surg 72A:355
16. Kudo H, Iwano K, Watanabe S (1980) Total replacements of the rheumatoid elbow with a hingeless prosthesis. J Bone Joint Surg 62A:277

17. Lowe LW, Miller AJ, Allum RK, Higginson DW (1984) The development of an unconstrained elbow arthroplasty: a clinical review. J Bone Joint Surg 66B:243
18. Morrey BF (1993) Revision of failed tatal elbow arthroplasty, the elbow and its disorders, 2nd edn. Saunders, Philadelphia, p 676
19. Morrey BF, Adams RA (1992) Semi-constrained arthroplasty for the treatment of rheumatoid arthritis of the elbow. J Bone Joint Surg 74A:479
20. Morrey BF, Bryan RS (1983) Infection after total elbow arthroplasty. J Bone Joint Surg 65A:330
21. Morrey BF, Bryan RS (1987) Revision total elbow arthroplasty. J Bone Joint Surg 69A:523
22. Morrey BF, Bryan RS, Dobyns JH, Linscheid RL (1981) Total elbow arthroplasty: a five-year experience at the Mayo Clinic. J Bone Joint Surg 63A:1050
23. Pritchard RW (1981) Long term follow-up study: semi-constrained elbow prosthesis. Orthopedics 4:151
24. Pritchard RW (1983) Anatomic surface elbow arthroplasty: a preliminary report. Clin Orthop 179:223
25. Roper BA, Tuke M, O'Riordan SM, Bulstrode CJ (1986) A new unconstrained elbow. J Bone Joint Surg 68B:566
26. Rosenberg G, Figgie HE III, Ranawat CS et al (1988) Total elbow replacement for rheumatoid arthritis. Long-term results with a semi-constrained prosthesis. Orthop Trans 12:732
27. Rosenberg GM, Turner RN (1984) Nonconstrained total elbow arthroplasty. Clin Orthop 187:154
28. Rozenfeld SR, Anzel SH (1982) Evaluation of the Pritchard total elbow arthroplasty. Orthopedics 5:713
29. Ruth JT, Wilde AH (1992) Capitellocondylar total elbow replacement. J Bone Joint Surg 74A:95
30. Rydholm U, Tjornstrand B, Petterson H, Lindgren L (1984) Surface replacement of the elbow in rheumatoid arthritis: early results with the Wadsworth prosthesis. J Bone Joint Surg 66B:737
31. Simmons ED, Sullivan JA, Ewald FC (1990) Long-term review of the capitellocondylar total elbow replacement. Orthop Trans 14:642
32. Soni RK, Cavendish ME (1984) A review of the Liverpool elbow prosthesis from 1974 to 1982. J Bone Joint Surg 66B:248
33. Souter WA (1981) A new appraoch to elbow arthroplasty. Engin Med 10:269
34. Trancik T, Wilde AH, Borden LS (1987) Capitellocondylar total elbow arthroplasty. Clin Orthop 223:175
35. Tuke MA (1981) The ICLH elbow. Engin Med 10:75
36. Verneuil A (1860) De la creation d'une fausse articulation par section ou resection partielle de l'os maxillarie inferieur, comme moyen de rededier l'anklylose orale de fausse de la machiore inferieur. Arch Gen Med 15:284
37. Volz RG (1982) Development and clinical analysis of a new semi-constrained total elbow prosthesis. In: Inglis AE (ed) Upper extremity joint replacement. Mosby St Louis
38. Wadsworth TG (1981) A new technique of total elbow replacement. Engin Med 10:69
39. Weiland AJ, Weiss A, Wills RP, Moore JR (1989) Capitellocondylar total elbow replacement. A long-term follow-up study. J Bone Joint Surg 71A:217
40. Wolfe SL, Figgie MP, Inglis AE et al (1990) Management of infection about total elbow prosthesis. J Bone Joint Surg 72A:198

Management of Problems Associated with Total Elbow Arthroplasty – Problems of Revision, Severe Bone Defect, Ulnar Nerve Neuropathy, and Total Elbow Arthroplasty for Fractured Elbow

H. Kudo

Revision of the failed total elbow arthroplasty (TEA) is generally a very difficult procedure, but the degree of difficulty depends very much on the cause or the nature of the failure. My experience with revision has been limited to patients who had previously undergone arthroplasty using our own prosthesis.

For the period of 10 years from 1972 to 1982, 39 operations with the type-1 or type-2 (Fig. 1) prosthesis were done in 38 patients at our hospital. As can be seen from Fig. 1, the type-2 prosthesis is a nonconstrained, surface replacement prosthesis; it should also be noted that the humeral component has no stem.

The intermediate and long-term results of the arthroplasty using these prostheses have already been published [1, 2], so it is unneccesary to go into detail about these results. I shall merely summarize the long-term results in brief.

The average follow-up time of this study was 9 years and 6 months. Among 37 elbows that could be followed up, a good result was seen in 29 elbows, a fair result in one, and a poor result in seven. Out of the seven elbows with a poor result, five needed revision because of gross posterior displacement of the humeral component.

Figure 2 shows an X-ray of the type-1 prosthesis 21 years after the operation. Although there is a moderate degree of subsidence of the humeral component, the clinical result of this elbow is still quite satisfactory.

Figure 3a shows gross posterior displacement of the humeral component. We had this type of failure in five elbows, four of which needed revision. We used a stemmed humeral component (type 3), for the revision of these elbows. Generally speaking, the revision was not difficult because a large amount of bone stock was still left in the humeral condyles. Figure 3b shows an X-ray 8 years after revision, the clinical result of this elbow is good.

In the chapter on "Cementless or Hybrid Total Elbow Arthroplasty" (this volume), I described our experience with the type-4 prosthesis, a cementless prosthesis made of titanium alloy, and referred to five elbows that needed revision. Figure 4a shows one of the five elbows which sustained a fracture at the base of the stem. Generally, the revision for these cases was not so easy, because the remaining portion of the broken stem was firmly fixed within the medullary canal. Figure 4b shows an X-ray after revision using a type-5 prosthesis made of cobalt-chromium alloy.

The next problem is how to manage elbows showing severe bone defect at the end of both the humerus and the ulna. Sometimes we see cases showing an almost

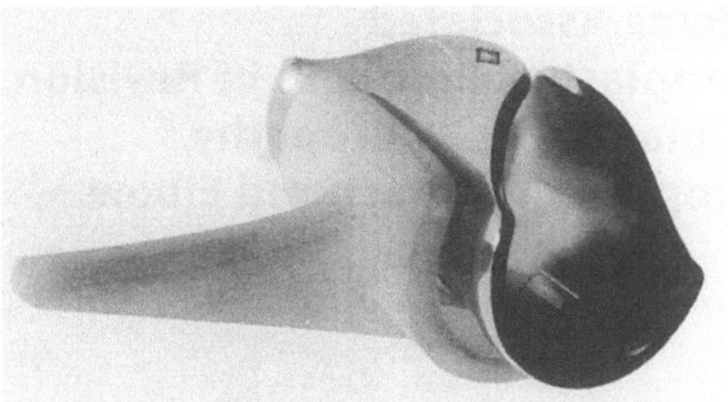

Fig. 1. Type-2 prosthesis

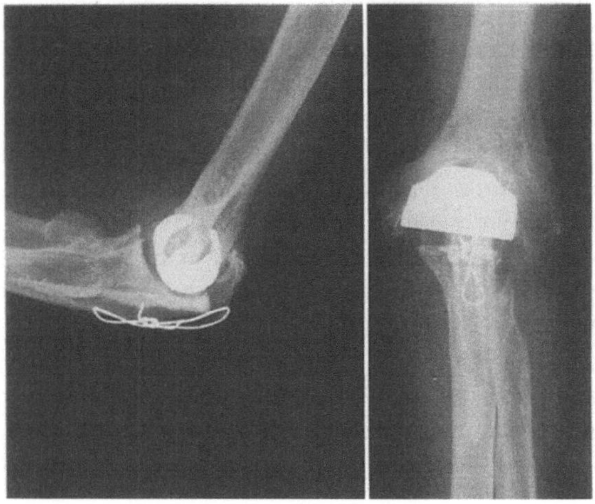

Fig. 2. Type-1 prosthesis 21 years after operation

complete defect of the medial humeral condyle in rheumatoid elbows, and in these cases the problems are not only pain, but also severe disturbance of function due to gross instability. As shown in Fig. 5a, for this type of elbow we have tried to reconstruct both the medial humeral condyle and the coronoid process of the ulna using a full-thickness iliac bone graft; Fig. 5b shows an X-ray of such an elbow before the operation and Fig. 5c an X-ray at $3\frac{1}{2}$ years after the operation. Fig. 6a,b shows the same type of elbow, and Fig. 6c,d shows an X-ray at $4\frac{1}{2}$ years after the operation. It seems that the bone grafting is effective and working well as a supporting bone block to the prosthesis.

Our next topic is ulnar nerve neuropathy. One of the commonest complications of total elbow arthroplasty is ulnar nerve paresis. However, in rheumatoid elbows, we often see cases with ulnar nerve paresis even before the operation due to entrapment by the pathology of rheumatoid arthritis.

In order to relieve preoperative neuropathy as well as to prevent the postoperative neuropathy which may occur as a complication, we have adopted a policy of extensive release of the ulnar nerve at the time of TEA.

From our experience we agree with the opinion of Dr. Gabel and Dr. Amadio [3] from Mayo Clinic in that the deep flexor/pronator aponeurosis which covers

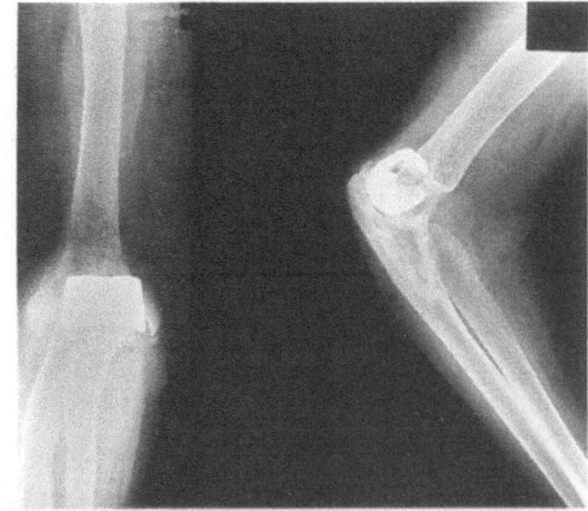

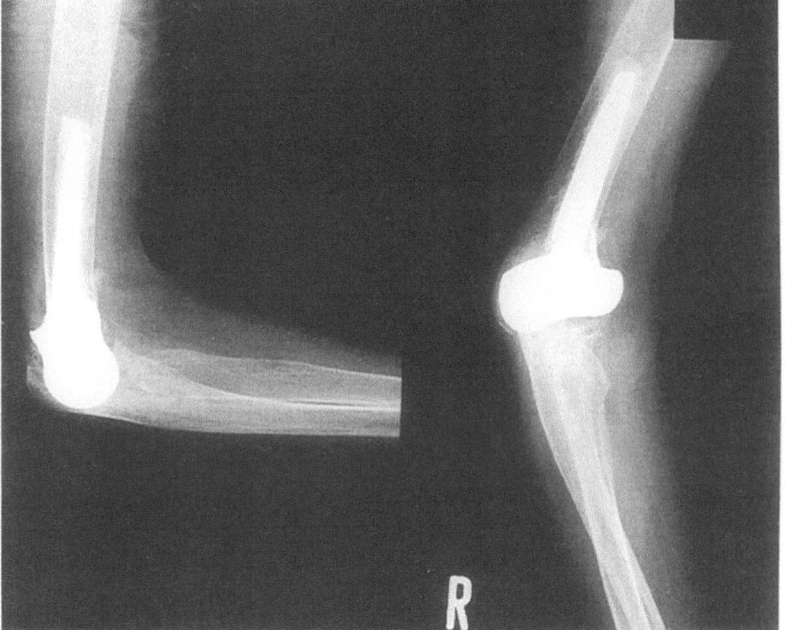

Fig. 3. a Gross posterior displacement of the humeral component. **b** 8 years after revision using a type-3 prosthesis

the nerve deep in the ulnar flexor muscle of the wrist may sometimes become the locus of entrapment.

So we feel it very important to release the nerve distally up to the level of the deep flexor–pronator aponeurosis.

Table 1 and Fig. 7 show the results of comparative measurement of the nerve conduction velocity performed consecutively for 1 year in the 14 elbows before and after TEA. When measured at 2 weeks after TEA, seven elbows showed a significant increase of the conduction velocity, six elbows showed no appreciable change, and in one elbow the conduction velocity could not be measured after the opera-

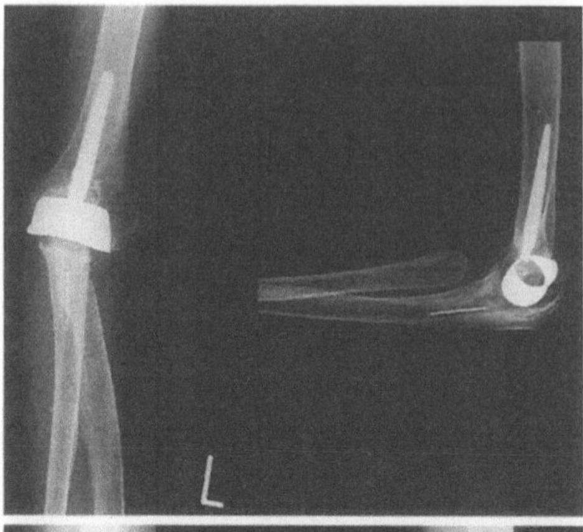

a

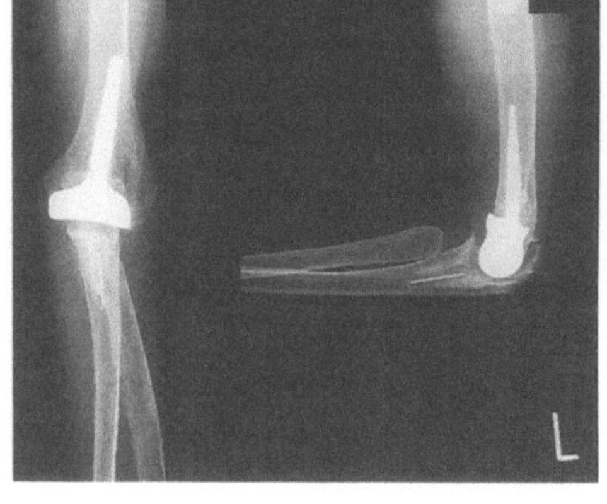

b

Fig. 4. **a** Fracture at base of stem. **b** Revision using a type-5 prosthesis

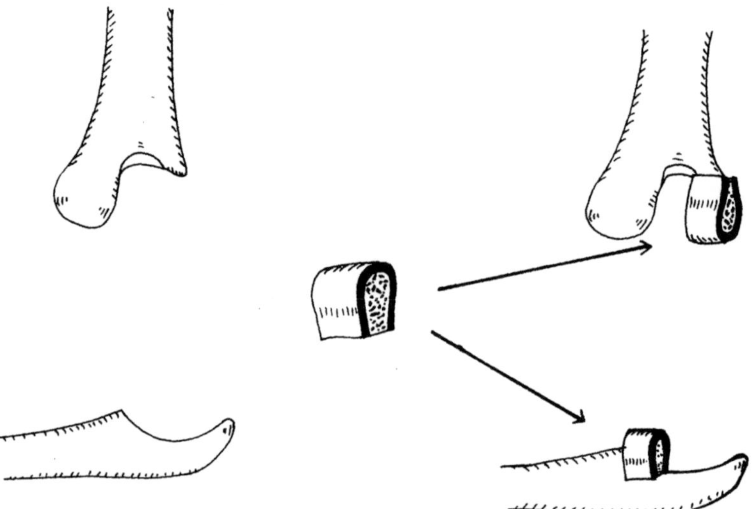

a

Fig. 5. **a** Reconstruction of the medial humeral condyle and the coronoid process of the ulna using a full-thickness iliac bone graft. **b** Before operation. **c** 3½ years after operation

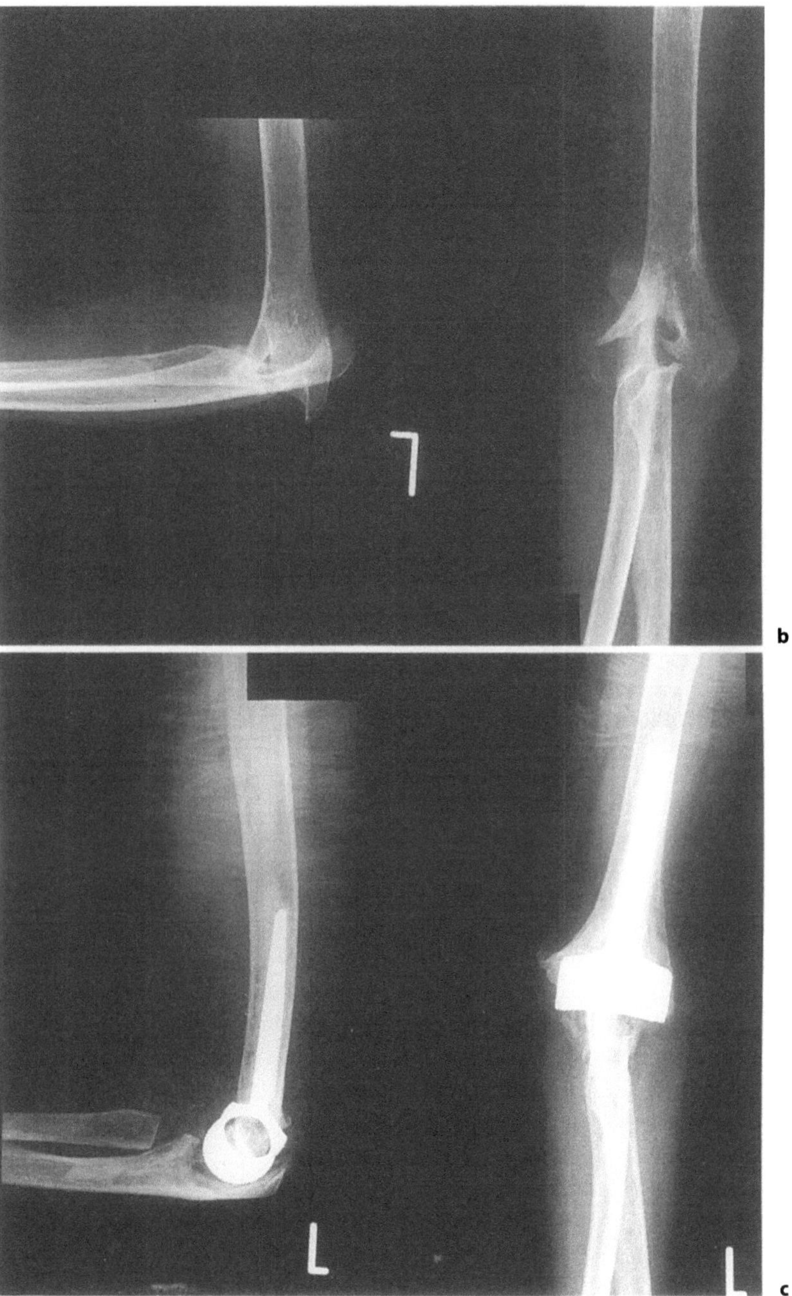

Fig. 5. b,c

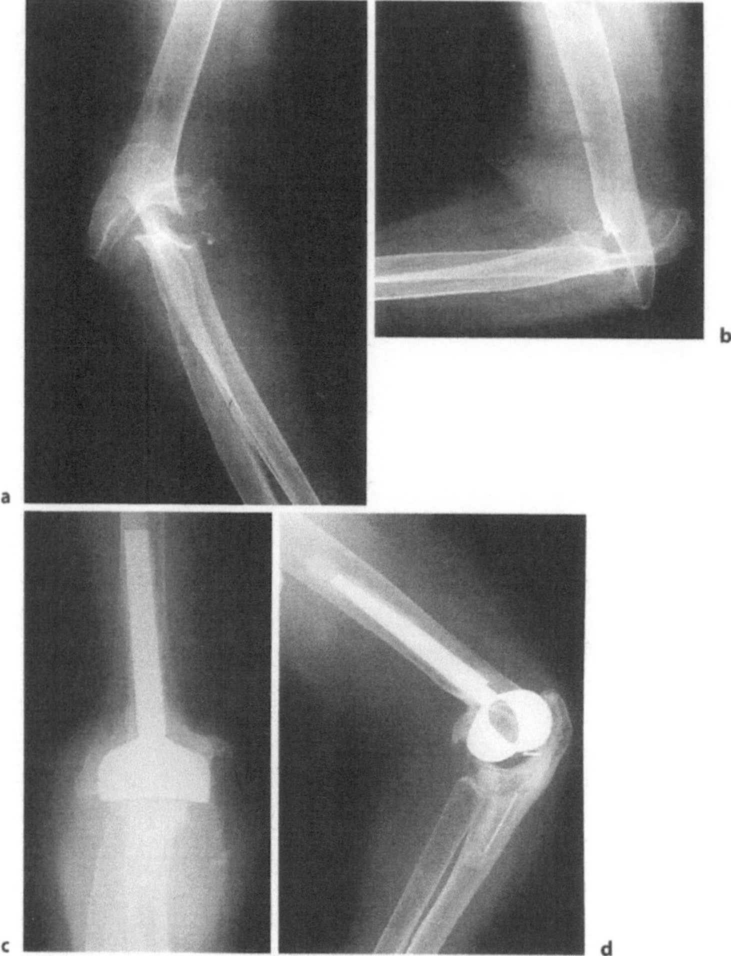

Fig. 6. a,b Same type of elbow as shown in Fig. 5. **c,d** 4½ years after operation

Table 1. Measurement of nerve conduction velocity

Preoperative	Postoperative			Total
	Increased	Unchanged	Unclear	
Normal	2	6	0	8
Slow	5	0	1	6
Total	7	6	1	14

Fig. 7. Comparative measurement of nerve conduction velocity

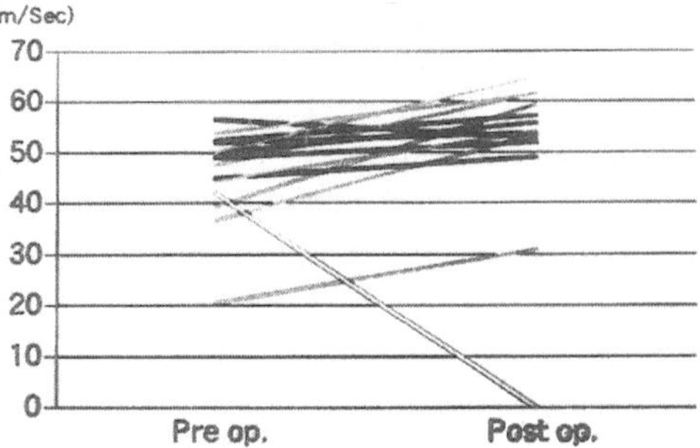

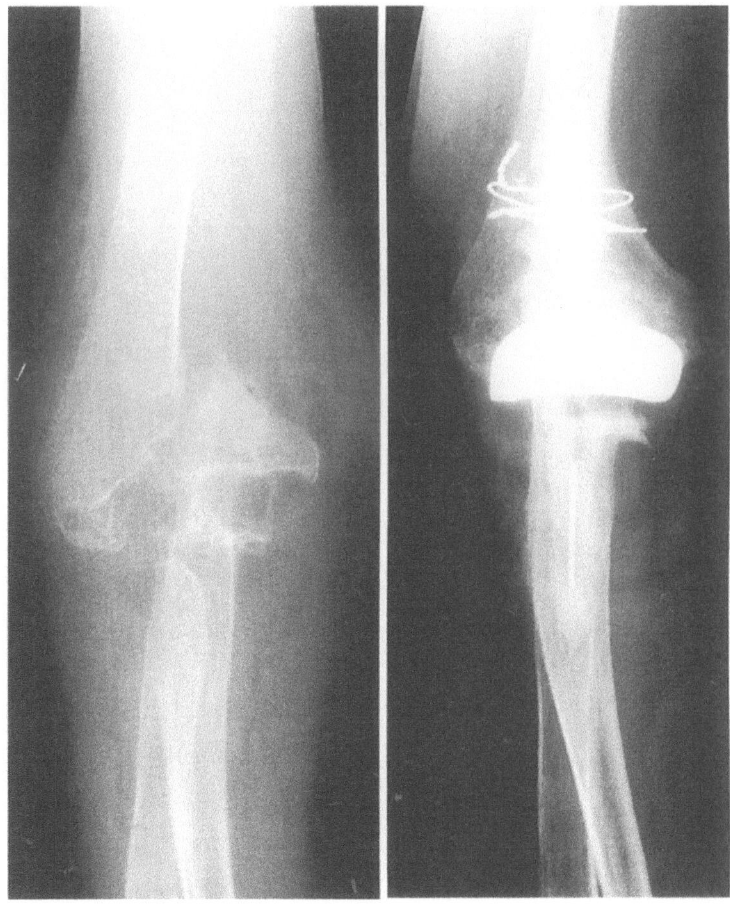

Fig. 8. a Periaticular fracture around elbow in partient with rheumatoid arthritis. **b** 5 years after total elbow prosthesis

tion for technical reasons. In the last case there had been nerve paresis before the operation; it was not clinically worsened, remaining unchanged after the operation.

Sometimes we encounter periarticular fracture around the elbow in patients with rheumatoid arthiritis. If the fractured elbow has already undergone severe erosive changes, one treatment option is the use of total elbow prosthesis.

Figure. 8a shows an X-ray of such a case in which the patient was treated by insertion of the prosthesis; Fig. 8b shows an X-ray at 5 years after the operation with solid union and good function of the elbow.

Figure 9a shows a case of comminuted T-fracture. TEA was performed, and Fig. 9b shows an X-ray at 5 years after the operation with a good result.

Figure 10a is a radiograph of an olecranon fracture. We did TEA in this case too, and the fragment of the olecranon was fixed by figure-of-eight wiring. Unfor-

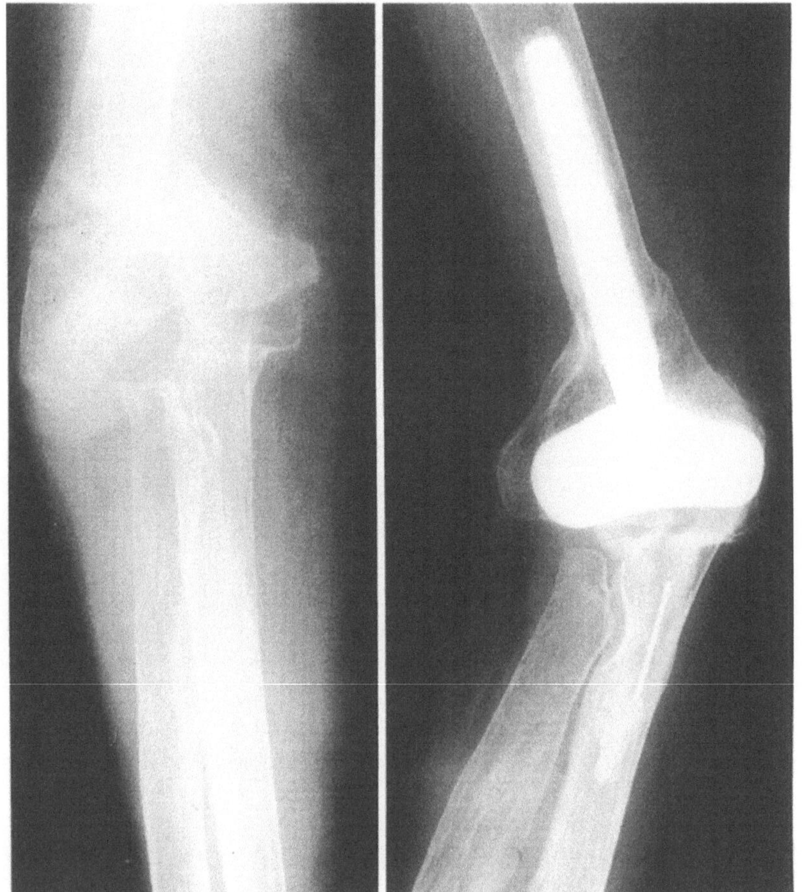

Fig. 9. a Comminuted T-fracture. **b** 5 years after total elbow arthroplasty

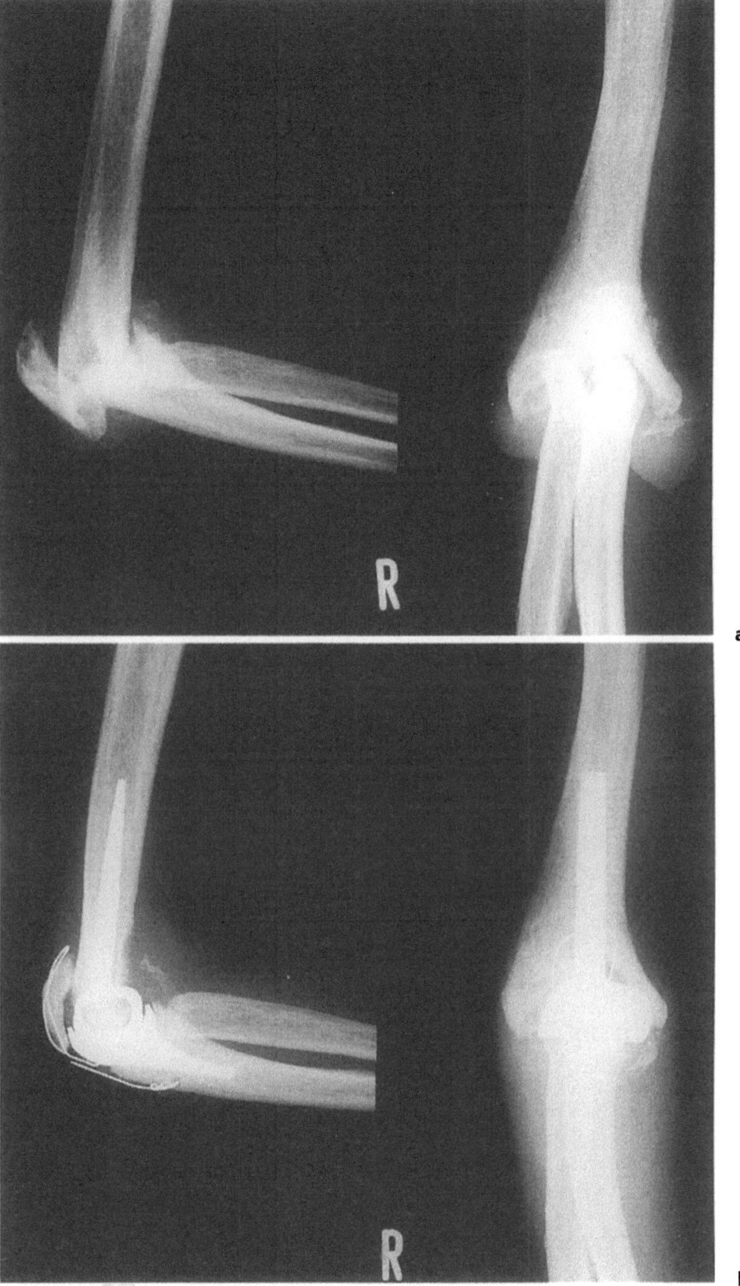

Fig. 10. Olecranon fracture. **b** Olecranon fixed by figure-of-eight wiring, but the wire broke. **c** Reoperation was performed to fix the fragment using a hook plate

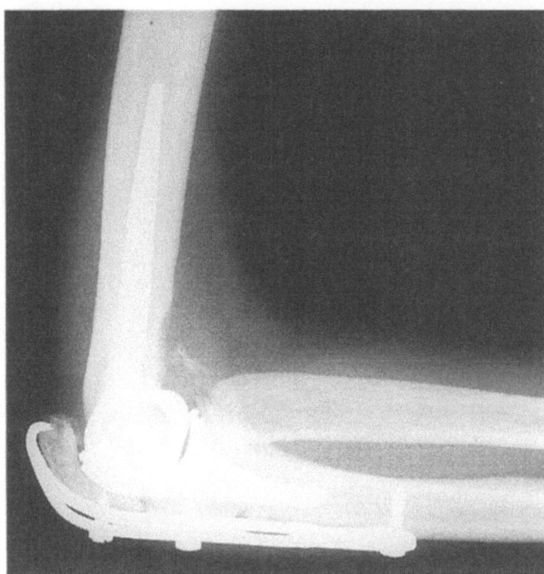

Fig. 10. c

tunately, the wire broke, as can be seen in Fig. 10b. We reoperated to fix the fragment using a hook plate (Fig. 10c). However, this is a recent case; we have to follow the future course carefully.

In summary, revision of a nonconstrained, surface-replacing prosthesis is easier and less risky because sufficient bone stock is still available. Severe defects of the medial humeral condyle can be managed by the use of nonconstrained, stemmed prosthesis and also by augmentation with autogenous bone block. Extensive release and anterior transfer of the ulnar nerve seems to be effective to prevent postoperative neuropathy. Intra-articular fracture around the elbow may better be treated by TEA in some patients with severe arthritis.

References

1. Kudo H, Iwano K, Watanabe S (1980) Total replacement of the rheumatoid elbow with a hingeless prosthesis. J Bone Joint Surg 62A:277
2. Kudo H, Iwano K (1990) Total elbow arthroplasty with a non-constrained surface-replacement prosthesis in patients who have rheumatoid arthritis; a long-term follow-up study. J Bone Joint Surg 72A:355
3. Gabel GT, Amadio PC (1990) Reoperation for failed decompression of the ulnar nerve in the region of the elbow. J Bone Joint Surg 72A:213

Complications After Capitellocondylar Elbow Replacement via the Lateral Approach

P. Ljung and U. Rydholm

Introduction

The capitellocondylar total elbow was developed in Boston some 20 years ago and has remained unchanged except for the addition of metal backing to the ulnar component. The prosthesis has been clinically used in Boston since 1974, and it was originally implanted through a posterior approach. The lateral, extended Kocher approach was adopted in 1979. In Lund, the capitellocondylar elbow has been used with the lateral approach since 1989. The lateral approach is of special interest, since the medial collateral ligament and the main part of the triceps tendon are left intact. Ewald et al. [2] reported that "the prevalence of complications was lower for the patients in whom the prosthesis had been implanted through the lateral approach than for those in whom it had been implanted through a posterior approach." There are few other reports in the literature on elbow replacement through the lateral approach.

Complications in prosthetic surgery of the elbow can be divided into major and minor ones. We define major complications as ones that threaten the survival of the prosthesis, e.g., deep infection, aseptic loosening, and dislocation. Minor complications include instability problems, wound healing complications, and ulnar nerve palsy. These complications are mostly transient and, perhaps because of that, often overlooked if not recorded prospectively.

Major Complications

Deep Infection

In the literature, the incidence of deep infection in prosthetic surgery of the elbow varies between 1% and 9%, with an average of 4–5%. There is no difference between different types of implants and no obvious tendency towards a lowered incidence in more recent reports. The incidence of deep infection following capitellocondylar elbow replacement via the lateral approach is low in the reports of Hodgson et al. [3] (none out of 23) and of Ewald et al. [2] (one out of 120) and in our own material (one out of 50).

Aseptic Loosening

Aseptic loosening is the major threat to the survival of the prostheses in the longterm. The rate of revision due to aseptic loosening is ten times higher for nonconstrained elbow prostheses without a humeral stem that for the capitellocondylar elbow, which is a cemented, resurfacing prosthesis with stemmed components. In fact, the rate of revision due to aseptic loosening of the capitellocondylar elbow is comparable to that of the hip and the knee.

Dislocation

In the short term, dislocation is considered to be the major problem with a nonconstrained elbow prosthesis; the overall incidence is 5%. With the lateral approach, the incidence is probably lower. We believe that dislocation can to a great extent be prevented by ensuring proper ligament and soft tissue tension, which is achieved by the use of ulnar components of varying thickness together with the lateral approach. Different ulnar components are tested against the intact medial collateral ligament in order to establish proper tension of the ligament. After cementation of the prosthesis, the lateral collateral ligament is resutured to the lateral epicondyle.

Minor Complications

Instability

Prosthetic instability, without dislocation, is of minor importance, since function is as a rule good and no adverse effects have been identified in the long term. With the capitellocondylar elbow, instability sometimes results in a lateral translocation of the ulnar component.

Wound Healing Complications

Delayed wound healing, wound hematoma, superficial infection, and wound breakdown are examples of wound healing complications. Wound healing problems are common following total elbow replacement, with an incidence of up to 30% and an average of 9%. Factors of importance for primary wound healing include diagnosis, previous surgery, medication with steroids and cytostatics, the size of the implant in relation to the thin soft tissue coverage, the surgical approach and extent of soft tissue dissection necessary, and the duration of postoperative immobilization. Some of these factors may give rise to wound healing complications as a consequence of impaired skin blood flow. Wound healing complications are of interest because they predispose to deep infection.

We have studied skin blood flow in the wound margins as a factor of importance for healing problems. Wound healing complications were registered prospectively in 50 capitellocondylar elbows in 42 patients with rheumatoid disease, five of which were investigated 1 day preoperatively and 2 days postoperatively with laser Doppler imaging (LDI). All elbows were operated on with a lateral approach. From the beginning of this series, the elbows were immobilized postoperatively for 5 days. As there were two cases of delayed wound healing among the first five elbows, the remaining 45 elbows were immobilized for 12 days. The five patients investigated with LDI were selected from the second group. LDI is a new technique with which a skin area of $12 \times 12\,\mathrm{cm}$ is scanned with a laser-Doppler instrument. Measurements from about 4000 points are obtained, processed in a computer, and presented as an image, where different blood flow values are represented by different colors in a scale from blue to red. Mean values from areas of interest can be calculated.

Postoperative immobilization has been reported to prevent wound healing complications following total elbow replacement [1, 4]. In our study, no wound healing complications were seen in the 45 elbows immobilized postoperatively for 12 days, but two cases of delayed wound healing were recorded for the five elbows immobilized for only 5 days. Factors other than the shorter postoperative immobilization time, such as the surgeons' learning curve, may have been of importance for the incidence of the two cases of wound complications, as they occurred early in our series, but the absence of wound complications in the 45 elbows immobilized for 12 days indicates that immobilization during wound healing is of importance to prevent healing problems. The outcome of the operation, in terms of range of motion, was not compromised by this postoperative regime. Mean extension was $-35°$ and mean flexion $145°$ with an average total range of motion of $110°$. Preoperative LDI in patients and controls showed no differences between their two elbows, but values in patients were higher than in controls, probably due to synovitis. Postoperative LDI values were considerably higher than preoperatively, which is expected in a situation of normal wound healing with unimpaired circulation of the wound margins. From this study, we can conclude that the rather extensive soft tissue dissection through the lateral approach does not compromise skin microcirculation and that 2 weeks of postoperative immobilization prevents wounds healing complications.

Ulnar Nerve Palsy

Ulnar nerve palsy is the most frequent complication of prosthetic surgery of the elbow, with a wide variation in severity, most cases being mild and transient. There is also a wide variation in reported incidence. The true incidence is certainly underestimated in retrospective studies, and comparisons between different studies are difficult to make. Ewald et al. [2] reported a decreased incidence of ulnar nerve problems in which the prosthesis had been implanted with the lateral approach compared to elbows in which a posterior exposure had been used, but

Hodgson et al. [3] reported a very high incidence of transient ulnar nerve palsy in laterally exposed elbows. We have recorded all complications prospectively and our experience is that transient ulnar nerve palsy is frequent following the lateral approach, but persistent ulnar nerve palsy is uncommon. Factors of importance for postoperative ulnar nerve palsy include rheumatoid ulnar neuropathy, compression of the ulnar nerve under the torniquet, neurolysis of the ulnar nerve with a possible damage of its vascular supply, direct injury to the nerve during surgery, compression of the nerve between the medial epicondyle and the olecranon or extensive stretching of the nerve during dislocation, and finally the possibility of heat injury during cement curing.

In an ongoing study, motor neurography of the ulnar nerve was performed during implantation of the capitellocondylar elbow through the lateral approach in order to identify critical moments during the operation. Four elbows in three patients with rheumatoid arthritis and one patient with osteoarthritis were investigated pre- and perioperatively. Preoperatively, sensory and motor neurography of the median and the ulnar nerves was performed bilaterally. Perioperatively, the ulnar nerve was repeatedly stimulated proximally, just distal to the axilla, and the amplitude of the compound muscle action potential from the abductor of the fifth finger was recorded distally. Bloodless field was not utilized and the ulnar nerve was not exposed. Preoperative ulnar nerve function was normal in all elbows, both electrophysiologically and clinically. Perioperative neurography showed the same pattern in all four elbows, with a reduction of amplitiude of compound muscle action potential at extreme dislocation of the elbow and normalization after relocation. Postoperative ulnar nerve function was clinically normal in all elbows. Our preliminary conclusion from this study is that extreme dislocation of the laterally exposed elbow carries a risk for ulnar nerve injury. The preventive effect of a release of the fibrous arch at the medial epicondyle has been suggested by Ewald et al. (1993) and is going to be tested in a forthcoming neurographic study. Our present philosophy is that the ulnar nerve should not be exposed if there is no history of preoperative neuropathy or of earlier surgical exposure. We believe that each surgical exposure of the ulnar nerve only adds further scarring with an increased risk for persistent neuropathy.

Concluding Remarks

Complications after nonconstrained elbow replacement could certainly be avoided to some degree. Deep infection is prevented by avoidance or early treatment of wound healing complications. Aseptic loosening is prevented by the use of cemented, condyle-supported, stemmed humeral components. Prosthetic dislocation and instability is prevented by the use of surgical techniques and prostheses that allows the surgeon to establish proper soft tissue tension. Wound healing complications can be prevented by postoperative immobilization during wound healing. Ulnar nerve palsy in laterally exposed elbows is prevented by reducing periods of extreme dislocation and perhaps by releasing the fibrous arch of the medial epicondyle.

We believe, from the complication point of view, that the lateral approach is an important part of the nonconstrained philosophy of the capitellocondylar elbow.

References

1. Brady O, Quinlan W (1993) The Guildford elbow. J Hand Surg 18-B:389–393
2. Ewald FC, Simmons ED, Sullivan JA, Thomas WH, Scott RD, Poss R, Thornhill TS, Sledge CB (1993) Capitellocondylar total elbow replacement in rheumatoid arthritis. J Bone Joint Surg 75-A:498–507
3. Hodgson SP, Parkinson RW, Noble J (1991) Capitellocondylar total elbow replacement for rheumatoid arthritis. J R Coll Surg Edinb 36:133–135
4. Maloney WJ, Schurman DJ (1989) Cast immobilization after total elbow arthroplasty. A safe cost-effective method of initial postoperative care. Clin Orthop 245:117–122

Elbow Reconstruction Using Cadaveric Allograft and an Elbow Endoprosthesis

D. Stanley

Introduction

Although much of the early work on bone transplantation and osteogenesis is accredited to the work of Judet, Axhausen and others [4], it was Sir William MacEwen [8] who, in 1909 in the *Annals of Surgery*, reported in his paper "Intra-Human Bone Grafting and Re-Implantation of Bone", a 30-year follow-up of this particular technique. He had used wedges of bone removed from children with Ricket's disease to reconstruct the humerus of a farmer who had been involved in a severe accident at work.

In 1925, Lexer [6] reported a 50% success rate following whole and partial joint allografts. Unfortunately, his long-term follow-up was incomplete. For several years after this, there was little interest in the technique, until improved methods of bone preservation were developed in the 1950s. This resulted in renewed interest in allografting, and several papers appeared during the 1970s reporting the results of this technique [6, 9, 13, 19]. Although some patients achieved long-term success, these authors noted that infection, graft non-union and fractures were the main problems associated with the procedure.

Ottolenghi [11] reported that in his experience partial joint allografts gave better results than when whole joint grafts were used.

More recently, there have been several reports showing the effectiveness of allografts for reconstruction around the hip [1, 2, 10] and also around the knee [14, 17].

The use of allografts in the upper limb has been less extensively studied. Urbaniak and Black [15] reported their experience with ten elbow allografts, of which eight were whole joint and two partial joint replacements. Although when their results were published, seven of the ten patients were considered to have satisfactory results, Urbaniak states that the long-term results were still unknown.

Since most of the recent reports on allografting in the lower limb have combined bone with an endoprosthesis, it was this technique that I have used at the elbow. This paper reports the results of three such cases, one following severe trauma to the lower end of humerus and the other two as a result of rheumatoid arthritis.

Allograft Types

Three types of allograft have been used for joint reconstruction, with most of the work being carried out in the lower limb for reconstruction of the hip and knee.

Whole Joint Allografts

The use of whole joint allografts involves implanting the whole joint together with its ligamentous supports. This type of procedure provides a physiological replacement, but unfortunately the longer-term results have been less satisfactory. With whole joint elbow allografts, Urbaniak reported significant complications such as non-union, instability and partial radial nerve injury. In addition, cartilage necrosis and subchondral bone collapse may occur with this type of joint replacement.

Partial Joint Allograft

The importance of an exact fit of the articular surface when partial joint allografts are used is believed to be essential [8, 12]. If the articular surfaces are not congruent, then cartilage necrosis, subchondral bone collapse and degenerative changes will occur. In addition, there will be a decreased range of normal joint movement.

Allograft Prosthesis Combination

Although there is little written on the subject of allograft prosthesis combination as regards elbow reconstruction, this technique is well documented in relation to hip and knee reconstruction [1, 2, 9, 10, 14]. It has been shown that the use of massive allografting enables large bone defects to be filled, restoring the bony architecture and reducing the need for custom-made prostheses.

Initial Preparation

Allografts are retrieved from donors aged between 18 and 60 years who have tested HIV (human immunodeficiency virus) negative. A clean retrieval is carried out within 48 h of death and then the distal humerus and proximal ulna are cleaned and processed in a class-100 environment.

This preparation procedure involves the removal of all soft tissue from the bone, after which the bone is packaged in polythene envelopes. Irradiation to 25 kGy is then performed and the allograft is stored at −70 °C until required.

Indications for Surgery

The three patients that we have treated with allograft prosthesis combination elbow replacements all presented with flail elbows. One rheumatoid patient had been referred, having previously undergone an elbow replacement. The ulna component had become loose and fractured through the proximal ulna.

The second case was another patient with rheumatoid arthritis who had fractured through the proximal ulna 2 years previously, with resultant proximal migration of the radius and ulna anterior to the distal humerus.

The third patient was a woman who, 12 months previously, had fallen, sustaining a distal comminuted humeral fracture together with an ipsilateral distal radius and ulna fracture. The fractures were treated with K-wire fixation and, although initially a satisfactory reduction was achieved, the K-wires in the humerus became loose and the patient went on to develop a pseudarthrosis of the distal humerus.

Preoperative Assessment

Before surgery, all patients underwent an infection screen in order to reduce the risk of infection developing at the elbow following reconstruction. In addition, patients who had undergone previous surgery had a preliminary drill biopsy performed with the specimens being sent for aerobic and anaerobic cultures. This was undertaken in order to reduce the potential risk of infection.

Surgical Technique

The surgical technique described is for those situations for which a distal humeral allograft is required. The important features of preparation for an ulnar allograft will be mentioned later.

The patient is placed in the lateral position with the affected arm uppermost and supported over a bolster. This allows the forearm to hang vertically and enables an excellent posterior exposure to the elbow joint.

The limb is exanguinated by elevation for several minutes prior to inflation of the tourniquet. A straight postero-medial incision is used and the ulnar nerve identified. The nerve is not mobilised, since it has been my experience that this can affect the blood supply and therefore the function of the nerve post-operatively. The nerve is, however, frequently observed during the operation and is at all times protected from injury. The triceps mechanism is then incised through its tendinous portion and elevated in continuity with the periosteum over the proximal ulna and olecranon. This envelope of tissue is reflected radially. The exposure is continued sufficiently distally in order that the radial head, maybe exposed and inspected. The radial head is then resected. Sufficient exposure is performed in order to facilitate dislocation of the joint.

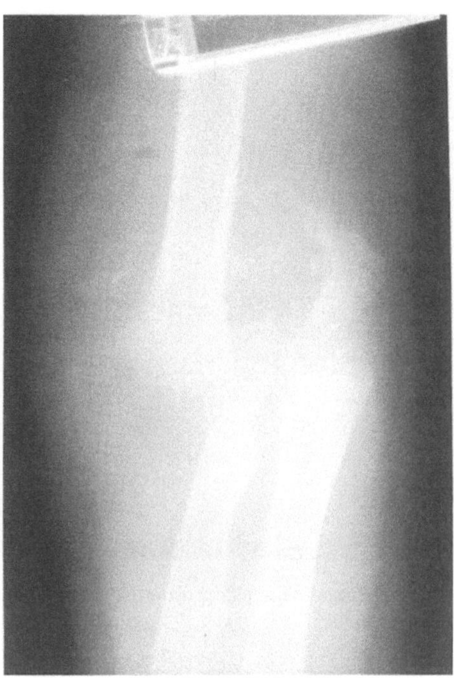

Fig. 1. Severe fracture of distal humerus with bone loss

At this point it is then possible to inspect the distal humeral damage, and only those bone fragments that do not have continuity with the shaft of the humerus are excised. Sometimes fragments of bone can be left with advantage if they are at the expected host – allograft junction. These fragments will then act as bone graft at the junctional zone. The humeral shaft is then prepared by opening up the intramedullary canal by resection of the distal humerus using a step cut. This cut is important, since when the allograft is finally prepared it will have an opposite step cut and this step gives some inherent rotational stability at the junctional zone. In addition, the step cut increases the surface area of the host allograft interface, thereby providing a greater area over which creeping substitution of host bone into allograft can occur. It is important that the minimum amount of host bone is resected in the preparation process.

When this stage is complete, the ulna should be prepared in just the same way as for a primary joint replacement.

While the patient's humerus and ulna preparation is proceeding, it is preferable for another team of surgeons to be preparing the allograft. The distal humeral allograft is cut and reamed in just the same way as for a primary joint replacement. At the end of the procedure the humeral implant should fit satisfactorily into the humeral allograft.

At this stage the humeral allograft should be aligned with the patient's humerus and it is at this stage that the final length adjustment is carried out. The length of allograft necessary to restore limb length can now be appreciated, and the

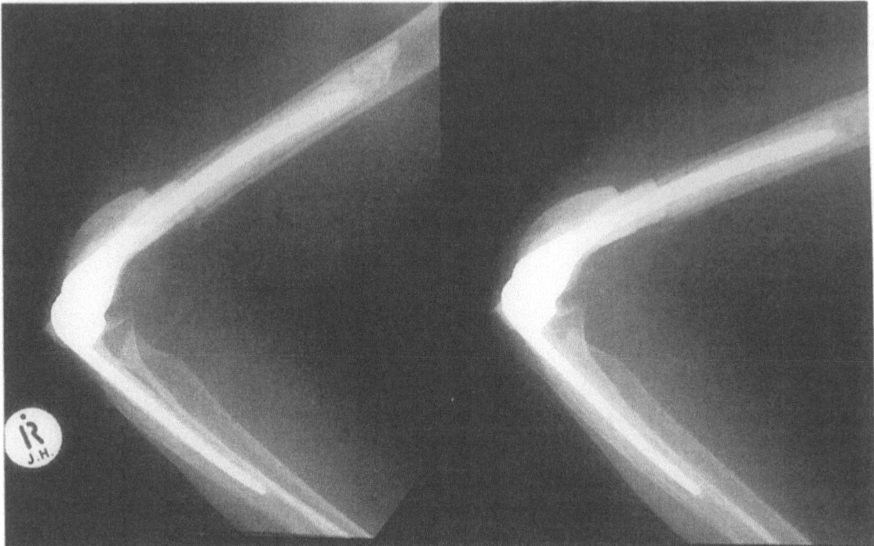

Fig. 2. Allograft and endoprosthesis: radiographs showing position immediately postoperatively and after 6 months

allograft should be marked using methylene blue so as to indicate the level of the step cut that will accurately interface with the host humerus. Having performed the step cut, the orientation should be checked and a trial reduction performed inserting the humeral component through the allograft and up into the host humerus. The ulnar component should be inserted and the two components linked together in order to check the soft tissue tension and range of elbow movement.

The component should then be removed, the tourniquet deflated and haemostasis achieved. The tourniquet is then once more re-inflated prior to cementing the components in place.

The humeral component is cemented into the allograft outside the body, leaving the stem of the implant projecting proximally from the bone. The allograft endoprosthesis is then cemented into the host humerus and at the same time the ulnar prosthesis is cemented in place. The components are linked together and the cement is allowed to harden. During fixation, it is important to be certain that there is no cement between the step cuts of the allograft and host bone. If this happens, it will affect the possibility of creeping substitution of bone from the host into the allograft bone.

Once the cement has hardened, bone graft is packed around the junctional zone, the tourniquet is deflated and final haemostasis achieved. The wound is closed over two Redivac drains, one being placed in the deep part of the wound and the other more superficially. Two drill holes are passed transversely through the olecranon in order to facilitate re-attachment of the extensor mechanism. The remainder of the wound is closed in a routine fashion. A compression dressing is applied together with an anterior plaster slab, which remains in place for 4 days. The drains are removed after 48 h.

The wound is inspected on the fourth day, the plaster slab removed and the patient allowed to gently flex and extend the elbow. Formal physiotherapy has not been found necessary in the three cases so far undertaken.

The preparation of ulnar allografts is carried out in a similar fashion, except that the step cut is performed in a different plane.

Patient Details

This allograft prosthesis technique has been undertaken in three patients, all women and all over the age of 70 at the time of presentation. Indeed, two patients were over 80 when surgery was undertaken. Each patient had presented with a flail arm and had no active flexion/extension movements. The patients with rheumatoid arthritis had suffered from the disease for more that 20 years and both had fractures at the elbow. In one patient, this was due to the rheumatoid arthritis, whilst in the other it was secondary to an elbow replacement which had failed.

Results

The results that are presented are my early experience with this technique. The minimum follow-up to date is 6 months and the longest 1 year. Having said this, however, each patient has now achieved active flexion and extension movements with the affected arm and has had a return of functional movements (patient 1, 16°–120°; patient 2, 45°–120°; patient 3, 60°–130°).

The only complication that occurred was a transient ulnar nerve palsy, and this was in the patient with rheumatoid arthritis who had sustained a fracture of the proximal ulna, with resultant migration of the radius and ulna, anterior to the distal humerus.

We have seen radiological evidence of creeping substitution occurring at the host–allograft interface.

Discussion

Deficient bone is often the major factor when considering the treatment options available for elbow salvage. Customised implants can be particularly useful in this situation, but difficulties can be experienced at operation if further bone resection is necessary or if the implant does not fit as expected.

The use of allografts for joint reconstruction have been shown to be of value around the hip [1, 2, 10], and around the knee [13, 14, 17]. The use of allografts around the elbow, however, has received less attention. Urbaniak and Black [15] reported their experience of cadaveric elbow allografts, but this study involved total elbow allografts in eight patients and distal humeral allografts in two patients. More recently, at the Seventh Congress of the European Society for Surgery of the Shoulder and Elbow, Faulkes [4] reported two cases of allograft salvage of failed total elbow arthroplasty.

In the three patients that have been presented here, the early results of allograft and prosthesis combinations appear to be very encouraging. The technique has allowed limb length restoration to be achieved and has provided support for the elbow endoprosthesis. Fixation of the allograft to the host has been obtained by intramedullary fixation, rather than the rigid screw and plate fixation methods advocated by Urbaniak. This approach was based on the work of Stockley, McCauley and Gross [14], who stated that multiple drill holes might produce vascular channels within the allograft and lead to vascularisation, with possible collapse of the graft. They preferred union of allograft to host bone to be achieved by creeping substitution at areas of contact.

This technique, whilst being clinically demanding and requiring appropriate bone banking facilities, may be of value for the treatment of patients with flail elbows, in whom significant bone stock has been lost. It is to be hoped that, with longer follow-up, this technique of elbow salvage will be shown to be as satisfactory as the similar procedures carried out around the hip and knee joints.

References

1. Allan DG, Lavoie GT, McDonald S, Oakeshott R, Gross AE (1991) Proximal femoral allografts in revisin hip arthroplasty. J Bone Joint Surg Br 73:235
2. Borja FS, Mnaymneh W (1985) Bone allografts in salvage of difficult hip arthroplasties. Clin Orthop 197:123
3. Chase SW, Herdon CH (1955) The fate of autogenous and homogenous bone grafts. A historical review. J Bone Joint Surg Am 37:809
4. Faulkes: Allograft salvage of failed total elbow arthoplasty. Proceedings of the seventh congress of the European Society for Surgery of the Shoulder and Elbow
5. Gross AE, Silverstein EA, Falk J, Falk R, Langer F (1975) The allotransplantation of partial joints in the treatment of osteoarthritis of the knee. Clin Orthop 108:7
6. Lexer E (1925) Joint transplantations and arthroplasty. Surg Gynecol Obstet 60:782
7. MacEwen W (1909) Intrahuman bone grafting and re-implantation of bone. Ann Surg
8. Mankin HJ, Doppelt SH, Sullivan TR, Tomford WW (1982) Osteoarticlar and intercalary allograft transplantaion in the management of malignant tumours of bone. Cancer 50:613
9. Mnaymneh W, Emerson RH, Borja F, Head WC, Malinin TI (1990) Massive allografts in salvage revisions of failed total knee arthroplasties. Clin Orthop 206:144
10. Oakeshott RD, Morgan DAf, Zukor DJ (1987) Revision total hip arthroplasty with osseous allograft reconstruction: a clinical and roentgenographic analysis. Clin Orthop 225:37
11. Ottolenghi CD (1972) Massive osteo and osteo-articular bone grafts. Technique and results of 62 cases. Clin Orthop 87:156
12. Rodrigo JJ (1983) The problem of fit in osteocartilaginous allografts. In: Friedlaender GD, Mankin HJ, Sell KW (eds) Osteochondral allografts: biology, baking and clinical applications. Little Brown, Boston, p 249
13. Samuelson KM (1988) Bone grafting and noncemented revision arthroplasty of the knee. Clin Orthop 226:93

14. Stockley I, McAuley JP, Gross AE (1992) Allograft reconstructionin total knee arthroplasty. J Bone Joint Surg Br 74:393
15. Urbaniak JR, Black KE (1985) Cadaveric elbow allografts. Clin Orthop 197:131
16. Volkov M (1970) Allotransplantation of joints. J Bone Joint Surg Br 52:49
17. Wilde AH, Schickendantz MS, Stulberg BN, Go RT (1990) The incorporation of tibial allografts in total knee arthroplasty. J Bone Joint Surg Am 72:815

Springer-Verlag and the Environment

We at Springer-Verlag firmly believe that an international science publisher has a special obligation to the environment, and our corporate policies consistently reflect this conviction.

We also expect our business partners – paper mills, printers, packaging manufacturers, etc. – to commit themselves to using environmentally friendly materials and production processes.

The paper in this book is made from low- or no-chlorine pulp and is acid free, in conformance with international standards for paper permanency.